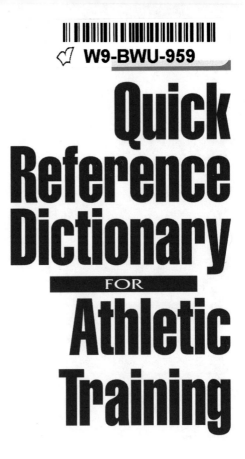

Quick
Reference
Dictionary

FOR

Athletic
Training

Quick Reference Dictionary

FOR

Athletic Training

Julie N. Bernier, EdD, ATC
Plymouth State College
Plymouth, NH

SLACK
INCORPORATED

An innovative information, education, and management company
6900 Grove Road • Thorofare, NJ 08086

The procedures and practices described in this book should be implemented in a manner consistent with the professional standards set for the circumstances that apply in each specific situation. Every effort has been made to confirm the accuracy of the information presented and to correctly relate generally accepted practices. The author, editor, and publisher cannot accept responsibility for errors or exclusions or for the outcome of the application of the material presented herein. There is no expressed or implied warranty of this book or information imparted by it.

The work SLACK publishes is peer reviewed. Prior to publication, recognized leaders in the field, educators, and clinicians provide important feedback on the concepts and content that we publish. We welcome feedback on this work.

Bernier, Julie
    Quick reference dictionary for athletic training / Julie Bernier.
        p. cm.
    Includes bibliographical references.
    ISBN 1-55642-461-2 (alk. paper)
    1. Physical education and training--Dictionaries. 2. Sports injuries--
Dictionaries. I. Title.

RC1206 .B475 2002
617.1'027'03--dc21

                                                            2002017748

Printed in the United States of America.
Published by: SLACK Incorporated
                     6900 Grove Road
                     Thorofare, NJ 08086 USA
                     Telephone: 856-848-1000
                     Fax: 856-853-5991
                     www.slackbooks.com

Contact SLACK Incorporated for more information about other books in this field or about the availability of our books from distributors outside the United States.

For permission to reprint material in another publication, contact SLACK Incorporated. Authorization to photocopy items for internal, personal, or academic use is granted by SLACK Incorporated provided that the appropriate fee is paid directly to Copyright Clearance Center. Prior to photocopying items, please contact the Copyright Clearance Center at 222 Rosewood Drive, Danvers, MA 01923 USA; phone: 978-750-8400; website: www.copyright.com; email: info@copyright.com.

For further information on CCC, check CCC Online at the following address: http://www.copyright.com.

Last digit is print number: 10   9   8   7   6   5   4   3   2   1

DEDICATION

This book is dedicated to my mentor and very good
friend David H. Perrin.

CONTENTS

ACKNOWLEDGMENTS

I wish to extend my sincere gratitude to the people at SLACK Incorporated, especially Amy McShane, Debra Toulson, Jill Tweedie, Michelle Gatt, and Olivia Lenahan. I especially want to thank Marge Albohm, who suggested I take on this project. My sincere thanks to Karen and Laela Jacobs and Jennifer Bottomley for providing the inspiration with the *Quick Reference Dictionary for Occupational Therapy* and *Quick Reference Dictionary for Physical Therapy*. I must thank my colleagues for putting up with me when I take on these projects and my students for inspiring me every day and reminding me why I came into this profession. I would like to thank the following students for their valuable input: Sara Lynn Gerhardt, Matthew Sartorio, and Krista Steckman. Lastly, I would like to thank the four most influential professionals in my life: Dr. David H. Perrin, Dr. Sherry Bovinet, Dr. Charlie Beach, and Dr. Dorothy Diehl.

ABOUT THE EDITOR

Julie N. Bernier, EdD, ATC is the department chair of the Health, Physical Education, and Recreation Department and director of graduate and undergraduate athletic training at Plymouth State College in Plymouth, NH, where she has been since 1988. Julie received her bachelor of science and master of education degrees from Keene State College in New Hampshire and doctorate from the University of Virginia. She serves on the editorial board of the *Journal of Athletic Training* and is a member of the NATA Research and Education Foundation Research Committee.

INTRODUCTION

This book is intended to serve as a reference tool for clinicians and students of athletic training. It provides quick reference to over 2100 terms related to the field of athletic training. Additionally, it contains 22 appendices that I hope you will find useful.

Appendices 1 to 3 were written to aid the practitioner or student in writing progress notes and includes a table of medical root terminology, acronyms and abbreviations, and symbols commonly used by practitioners. Appendices 4 through 11 serve as an anatomical reference for the student; Appendix 4 includes anatomical terms; Appendix 5 provides figures of the superficial and deep muscles of the body followed by a table that includes origin, insertion, action, and nerve innervations. Appendix 6 provides a table of normal joint ranges of motion. Appendix 7 provides a review of cranial nerves; Appendix 8 includes information on grading systems for assessment of concussion, while Appendices 9 through 12 cover nerve root assessment and peripheral nerve innervations. Appendices 13 through 15 provide assessment scales for muscle grading, grades of pain, and normal and abnormal end feels. The most comprehensive section, Appendix 16, provides information for more than 85 orthopedic special tests. Finally, Appendices 17 through 22 provide quick access to pertinent NATA membership information such as the NATA Code of Ethics, NATA Membership Policies and Privileges, NATABOC Standards of Professional Practice, and NATABOC State Licensure Boards.

A

Aβ: An afferent nerve fiber that is stimulated by touch, pressure, tension, movement, and vibration.

A δ fiber (A delta): An afferent neuron responsible for carrying temperature and noxious stimuli; responsible for "fast pain."

abdomen, acute: Acute onset of abdominal pain due to any number of causes including appendicitis, cholecystitis, perforated ulcer, and ruptured spleen.

abdominal aneurysm: An aneurysm within the abdomen. *See* aneurysm.

abdominal cavity: The cavity formed between the abdominal wall and the spine that houses a number of organs including the stomach, colon, small intestine, liver, gallbladder, pancreas, spleen, kidneys, bladder, and rectum.

abdominal guarding: Involuntary contraction of the abdominal muscles to protect organs in response to injury or illness to one or more organs.

abdominal quadrants: Four parts or divisions of the abdomen determined by drawing imaginary vertical and horizontal lines through the umbilicus. The upper left quadrant contains the stomach, spleen, and pancreas; upper right contains the liver and gallbladder; lower right contains the appendix; and lower left contains the colon.

abducens nerve: Cranial nerve VI; innervates the lateral rectus femoris muscle of the eye, responsible for lateral eye movement. *See* Appendix 7.

abduct: To move away from the midline in the frontal plane.

abduction (ABD): Movement of a body part (usually the limbs) away from the midline of the body.

abductor muscle: A muscle whose primary responsibility is to abduct the limb.

abrasion: Minor wound in skin surface, caused by rubbing or scraping.

abscess: Collection of pus.

absolute refractory period: The period following depolarization in which another action potential cannot occur.

absorption: The taking in of liquids, gases, or light.

AC joint (acromioclavicular joint): The articulation between the acromion process (the distal end of the spine of the scapula) and the lateral end of the clavicle. The acromioclavicular ligament forms the capsular ligament while the trapezoid and conoid ligaments (coracoclavicular ligaments) strengthen this articulation.

AC shear test: AC joint compression test. Test to examine the integrity of the AC joint. *See* Special Tests—Shoulder (Appendix 16).

acceleration: The change in velocity per unit of time (meters per second per second—m/s^2). For example, 1 m/s^2 means that velocity is increased by 1 m/s every second. *See also* gravity.

accessory motion: The small motions of sliding, spinning, and rolling that are necessary in order to have physiological motion.

accessory movers: Muscles that assist the prime movers in performing a function.

accessory nerve: Cranial nerve XI responsible for the innervation of the sternocleidomastoid and the trapezius muscles. *See* Appendix 5.

acclimatization: To adapt to a new temperature, climate, environment, or situation; the act of adapting to altitude, usually taking 1 to 3 days for each change in altitude.

accommodating resistance: As in the resistance given by an isokinetic dynamometer. The resistance supplied by the dynamometer is equal to the resistance put in by the patient.

accommodation: Adaptation, adjustment, the act of adjusting to a stimulus.

ACE inhibitor: A drug that inhibits the formation of angiotensin II; used to treat high blood pressure.

acetabulum: The "cup-shaped" socket of the hip joint that articulates with the head of the femur.

acetaminophen: A pain-relieving drug commonly known as Tylenol.

acetylsalicylic acid: Aspirin; a nonsteroidal anti-inflammatory used for the relief of pain and fever.

achalasia: A disease of the esophagus in which the ability to swallow is impaired.

Achilles' tendon: The distal insertion of the gastrocnemius and soleus muscles into the plantar surface of the calcaneus; Syn: calcaneal tendon.

ACI: *See* approved clinical instructor.

acid reflux: A condition in which stomach acid enters the esophagus.

acid-base balance: Refers to the control of pH in which the body's fluids are neither acid nor alkaline.

acidosis: An abnormal condition in which the pH is too low (ie, becomes acidic); caused by diabetes, kidney, or lung disease; leads to ketoacidosis in the diabetic individual.

acne vulgaris: A skin condition that most commonly affects adolescents; characterized by pus-filled pimples on the skin caused by overactivity of the oil glands.

acquired: A condition not contracted at birth but one that later develops.

acquired immunodeficiency syndrome (AIDS): Disease of the immune system caused by the human immunodeficiency virus (HIV).

acromegaly: A disease in which there is continued production of growth hormone by the pituitary gland after the end of adolescence.

acromion: The distal end of the spine of the scapula that forms the top of the shoulder.

acromion process: The superior lateral process of the spine of the scapula that articulates with the clavicle and forms the "top" of the shoulder.

acromioplasty: The surgical removal of the inferior distal end of the acromion process of the scapula; a procedure used to relieve soft tissue impingement in the subacromial space.

action potential: The change in voltage across the membrane of nerve or muscle.

active assistive range of motion (AAROM): Movement at a joint achieved by muscular contraction of the agonist muscles with assistance.

active electrode: In electrical stimulation, in which a monopolar pad placement is used (two pads of unequal size), it is the smaller of the two pads placed over the injured site, trigger point, motor point, or nerve.

active range of motion (AROM): Movement at a joint achieved by muscular contraction of the agonist muscles.

activities of daily living (ADLs): The skills required for independence in everyday living including activities such as mobility and self-care.

acuity test, visual: A test to measure the clarity of vision; *See also* Snellen's chart.

acupressure: Pressure applied to trigger points or acupuncture points with the intent of pain control.

acupuncture: An ancient Asian healing therapy employing the use of long, very fine needles, used in modern times as a method of pain control.

acute: Referring to brief exposure, sudden, of short duration, not chronic; sometimes used to mean severe.

acute mountain sickness (AMS): *See* altitude sickness.

acute otitis media: Inflammation of the middle ear.

acute respiratory disease: A life-threatening emergency in which O_2 levels drop and breathing becomes labored.

adaptation: Accommodation, to adjust to a stimulus.

addiction: A condition in which individuals cannot control their desire for alcohol, tobacco, food, exercise, or other activities.

Addison's disease: Chronic insufficiency of the adrenal cortex characterized by skin discoloration, anemia, weakness, and low blood pressure. Tuberculosis is the cause of approximately 20% of cases.

adduct: To move toward the midline in the frontal plane.

adduction (ADD): Movement toward the midline.

adenitis: Inflammation of the lymph nodes.

adenoidectomy: The surgical removal of the adenoids.

adenoids: Lymph tissue found in the superior aspect of the throat.

adenosine triphosphate (ATP): Adenine, ribose, and triphosphate (three phosphates) that store energy which is released when ATP is split into ADP (diphosphate) or AMP (monophosphate).

adhesion: The union of tissue surfaces, also referring to the formation of scar tissue that often occurs following surgery.

adhesive capsulitis: Also known as "frozen shoulder"; a condition in which scarring occurs in the shoulder joint capsule, a complication of rotator cuff injury or bursitis.

adipose tissue: A term for "fatty tissue"; tissue composed mainly of fat cells.

adjuvant: From the Latin term *adjuvans* meaning "to help" or "to reach a goal"; adjuvant therapy is a form of treatment that increases the effect of a drug or increases the likelihood of a positive outcome.

adrenal gland: An endocrine organ that lies anteromedial to the kidneys and is responsible for production of glucocorticoid, mineralocorticoid, androgenic hormones, epinephrine and norepinephrine.

adrenaline: Also known as epinephrine; a naturally occurring substance produced in the medulla of the adrenal gland; its release is part of the "fight-or-flight" response in which there is a dilation of blood vessels and an increase in heart rate and strength of contractions.

Adson's maneuver: A special test of the shoulder specifically for thoracic outlet syndrome. *See* Special Tests—Shoulder (Appendix 16).

adult-onset diabetes: *See* type II diabetes.

advance medical directives: Living will, durable power of attorney for health care, and health care proxy are examples of advance medical directives; instructions related to the treatment desires of an individual who cannot speak on his or her own behalf.

adverse effect: *See* adverse reaction.

adverse reaction: A negative or unwanted effect of a treatment.

aerobic training: Exercise that provides cardiovascular overload so as to develop functional capacity of the circulatory system and enhance aerobic capacity of specific muscles.

aesthesiometer: A device used to measure cutaneous sensitivity or the level of anesthesia. A two-point discriminator is an example of an aesthesiometer.

aetiology: *See* etiology.

affective disorder: A psychological condition in which the individual suffers extremes in moods and emotions; seasonal affective disorder (SAD) is an illness in which the individual is affected by the shorter days and lack of natural light during the fall and winter.

afferent: Conducting toward the center. In the case of nerves, conducting toward the brain, responsible for bringing sensory information to higher centers.

agenesis: The underdevelopment or nondevelopment of an organ or projection.

agonist: Muscle or muscle group responsible for a given joint motion. Its opposite is the antagonist.

AIDS: *See* acquired immunodeficiency syndrome.

AIDS-related complex: Symptoms related to HIV.

air embolism: Caused during surgery or from injury, it is the presence of air in the arteries that can cause a blockage.

airway obstruction: Anything that inhibits the passage of air to the lungs.

akinesia: Impaired body movement; absence of movement.

akinetic: Literally means "without movement"; refers to impaired, deficient, or lack of movement.

albinism: A disorder in which there is a reduction in melanin which is responsible for the pigment of hair, skin, and eye color.

albumin: A water-soluble protein responsible for the maintenance of plasma volume.

alcoholic cardiomyopathy: Heart damage or heart failure caused by the consumption of alcohol.

aldosterone: A hormone responsible for the regulation and balance of sodium and water in the body.

alimentary canal: The digestive tract.

alkalosis: A high pH; an abnormal condition in which there is a decrease in the normal acidity of the blood resulting from the accumulation of base or the depletion of acid. Can be caused by dehydration due to vomiting, hyperventilation, or high altitudes.

Allen's test: A special test of the shoulder used to assess thoracic outlet syndrome. *See* Special Tests—Shoulder (Appendix 16).

allergen: A substance that causes an allergic reaction.

allergic rhinitis: A reaction to a substance causing sneezing, runny nose, and sore eyes.

allograft: A transplant of tissue between allogeneic individuals (ie, a member of one's own species).

all-or-none response: A principle in which the depolarization of a membrane requires a minimum intensity to reach threshold. Once threshold is met, depolarization occurs to the fullest extent. An increase in intensity has no increased effect.

alopecia: Baldness; alopecia areata is characterized by patchy bald spots; alopecia capitis totalis is total loss of hair.

alpha level: The probability of chance occurrence. The alpha level is chosen *a priori.*

alprenolol: A beta-blocker used to treat high blood pressure, angina, and arrhythmias of the heart.

ALS: *See* amyotrophic lateral sclerosis.

alternating current (AC): A current that reverses its polarity; a current that crosses the isoelectric line; *see also* biphasic current.

alternative medicine: Holistic medicine; treatment methods not scientifically proven and generally not practiced in traditional medical facilities.

altitude sickness: An illness that affects nearly three-quarters of all people ascending to heights over 8000 feet. Symptoms include headache, dizziness, and nausea. The reduced air pressure can cause fluid to collect around the lungs and brain. If acclimatization does not occur, altitude illness can lead to a life-threatening condition.

alveolitis: Inflammation of the alveoli can progress to fibrosis or emphysema.

Alzheimer's disease: The most common form of dementia; it is a progressive disorder of the brain that first appears late in life and is characterized by memory loss, confusion, and a continued physical decline; marked by a degeneration of neurons in the cerebral cortex and the presence of beta-amyloid plaques. Named for Alois Alzheimer (1864-1915), a German neurologist who published a description of arteriosclerotic atrophy of the brain in 1894.

ambulation: The act or moving freely; walking.

ambulatory care: Outpatient care.

amenorrhea: The absence of the menstrual period for more than 3 months in women who had previously experienced menstruation and are not pregnant.

amine: A nitrogen compound derived from ammonia.

amino acid: A protein-building block.

amnesia: The loss of or impairment of memory: Anterograde is a loss of memory of events occurring after the injury; retrograde is a loss of memory of events occurring prior to the injury.

amniocentesis: A procedure in which a small amount of amniotic fluid is removed from the mother's womb for testing of potential fetal disorders.

ampere (A): Unit of electrical current, abbreviated as amps; SI unit of electrical current, equal to the flow of 1 volt through or resistance of one ohm.

amplitude: Magnitude, intensity; depicted by the height of the waveform.

amyotrophic lateral sclerosis (ALS): Also known as Lou Gehrig's disease; a progressive disease of the motor neurons in which function is gradually lost.

anabolic steroid: A group of usually synthetic hormones that increase constructive metabolism. Anabolic steroids are frequently abused in sports that require strength and size.

anaerobic exercise: Activity in which the body incurs an oxygen debt; exercise occurring in the absence of oxygen.

analgesia: A state in which there is a reduction of or an inability to feel pain.

analgesic: A pharmacological agent designed to reduce pain.

analysis of covariance (ANCOVA): A statistical procedure designed to account for the influence of one or more variables that correlate.

analysis of variance (ANOVA): A statistical procedure used to establish whether a statistically significant difference exists between two or more samples.

anaphylaxis: A histamine reaction to an allergen. Can result in a severe systemic reaction including edema, circulatory failure, and death.

anastomosis: A communication between vessels or organs that are normally not connected; a surgical procedure in which a connection is made between healthy sections of the colon or rectum after a cancerous or diseased portion has been removed.

anatomical position: A reference position in which the body is upright, all joints are extended to the neutral position, and palms are facing forward.

anatomical snuffbox: A hollow on the radial aspect of the wrist when the thumb is extended caused by the tendons of the extensor pollicis longus and brevis. The name originates from the use of this space to hold powdered "snuff" tobacco.

anatomy: The study of body structure.

androgen: A male sex hormone that produces male sex characteristics.

anemia: Reduced hemoglobin; symptoms include fatigue, and decreased resistance to infection.

anesthesia: Decreased sensation caused by neurological dysfunction or pharmacological agent.

aneurysm: A bulge in the wall caused by localized dilatation of an artery, vein, or the heart.

angioplasty: The use of surgery to make a damaged blood vessel function properly again; may involve widening or reconstructing the blood vessel.

Angiotensin-converting enzyme (ACE): A vasoconstricting peptide.

angina pectoris: Pain experienced in the chest, arms, or jaw because of a lack of oxygen to the heart muscle.

angle of pull (of a muscle): The angle formed by a longitudinal line through the bone from the axis and through the line of action (line of pull) of the muscle.

anisocoria: Unequal pupil size.

anisotropic: Having different mechanical properties depending upon direction of the load or force of application.

ankle-foot orthosis (AFO): A prosthetic for the foot or ankle; an AFO is commonly used for "drop-foot syndrome."

ankle mortise: The ankle joint; talocrural joint; the articulation between the tibia and the talus.

ankylosing spondylitis: Rheumatic disease of the synovial joints of the vertebrae. In severe cases, the spine becomes completely fused.

ankylosis: A disease process that results in the stiffening or fusion of a joint.

annulus fibrosis: The tough outer covering of a vertebral disk.

anode: The positive electrode. The electrode toward which negatively charged ions are attracted.

anomaly: A deviation from the norm.

anorexia nervosa: Most common in females, loss of appetite most commonly caused by an obsession to lose weight. Symptoms can be severe and can cause death.

anosmia: The loss of the sense of smell, often due to obstruction of the airway or injury to the olfactory nerve.

ANOVA: *See* analysis of variance.

anoxia: Decreased oxygen to the tissues, occurs frequently at high altitude.

antacid: A pharmacologic agent used to counteract the effects of hydrochloride acid released during digestion. Common agents include sodium bicarbonate, magnesium hydroxide, aluminum hydroxide, and calcium carbonate.

antagonist: The muscle or muscle group responsible for producing motions opposite of that being performed. The opposite of agonist.

anterior apprehension test: A special test of the shoulder to assess the anterior stability of the glenohumeral joint. *See* Special Tests—Shoulder (Appendix 16).

anterior cruciate ligament (ACL): A major ligament of the knee that prevents forward displacement of the tibia from the femur. The term cruciate literally means "to cross" and refers to the "crossing position" of the anterior and posterior cruciate ligaments. Females are two to eight times more likely to suffer ACL injury than males.

anterior draw (drawer) test: A special test of the knee to assess the continuity of the anterior cruciate ligament or of the ankle to assess the anterior talofibular, deltoid, and anterior tibiofibular ligaments. *See* Special Tests—Knee, and Ankle (Appendix 16).

anteroposterior: From anterior to posterior.

anteversion: A forward displacement. An anteverted hip is characterized by increased medial rotation.

anthropometry: The science involved in measurement and comparison of the human body.

antibiotic: A pharmacologic agent used to treat infections by inhibiting the growth of microorganisms.

antibody: A protein that is part of the immune response that is produced by white blood cells in response to a foreign protein.

anticoagulant: A substance that hinders coagulation.

antiemetics: A pharmacologic agent used to treat nausea and vomiting.

antihistamine: A pharmacologic agent used to treat allergic reactions by inhibiting the effects of histamine.

antihypertensives: A pharmacologic agent used to treat high blood pressure.

anti-inflammatory: An agent used to reduce inflammation.

antioxidants: A substance that protects cells from oxygen free radicals.

antipruritic: A pharmacologic agent used to reduce itching.

antipsychotic: A pharmacologic agent used to treat severe mental disorders.

antipyretic: A pharmacologic agent used to reduce fever.

antiseptic: A bacteria-killing chemical used to prevent infections by its application on the skin.

anus: The opening at the distal end of the rectum.

aorta: The main artery leaving the heart responsible for supplying oxygenated blood to the body.

apex: The tip, or most superior portion, of a tissue.

aphasia: A disease of the left brain in which both speech and understanding of speech are affected.

aplasia: The complete or partial failure of any organ or tissue to grow.

aplastic anemia: A condition in which there is reduction in the number of red blood cells, white blood cells, and platelets.

Apley's compression: A special test of the knee used to assess the meniscus. *See* Special Tests—Knee (Appendix 16).

Apley's distraction: A special test of the knee used to differentiate between injuries to the meniscus and ligament injury. *See* Special tests—Knee (Appendix 16).

Apley's grind test: *See* Apley's compression.

Apley's scratch test: A special test of the shoulder used to determine range of motion. *See* Special Tests—Shoulder (Appendix 16).

apnea: A period where breathing stops.

aponeurosis: A fibrous sheath continuous with muscle fibers giving rise to the origin and insertion, in some cases becoming a tendon.

apophysis: A bony outgrowth.

apparent leg length: A leg length measurement taken from umbilicus to medial malleolus, useful only when true (real) leg length differences are negative. A positive test is indicative of pelvic obliquity.

appendectomy: The surgical removal of the appendix.

appendicitis: Inflammation of the appendix.

appendicular skeleton: The upper and lower extremities.

appendix: A small, finger-like projection of the large intestine.

apprehension test: A special test which by its nature causes the patient to become apprehensive or withdraw, especially when the sensation of dislocation is imminent; patella apprehension, anterior, posterior, and inferior (shoulder) apprehension.

approved clinical instructor (ACI): A certified athletic trainer who has successfully completed an ACI workshop conducted by the clinical instructor educator from the institution in which the ACI will be supervising athletic training students. In order to assess clinical proficiencies of a student enrolled in a Commission on Accreditation of Allied Health Education Programs (CAAHEP) accredited program, one must be an ACI.

approximate: To bring near, to place next to; the act of bringing the edges of a wound together.

approximation test: A special test used to assess sacroiliac dysfunction in which the patient is positioned side-lying, and the examiner applies a downward pressure of the iliac crest.

arch: A bony structure that resembles an arch and imparts elasticity or flexibility to it; the foot has four main arches. The medial longitudinal arch, the long arch of the foot, is made up of the tuberosity of the calcaneus, talus, navicular, cuneiforms, and the heads of the first three metatarsals and is supported by the plantarcalcaneon-avicular ligament, the plantar fascia, and the intrinsic and extrinsic muscles and tendons of the foot. The lateral longitudinal arch is made up of the calcaneus, cuboid, and fourth and fifth metatarsals and is supported by the peroneals, abductor digiti minimi, flexor digitorum brevis, the long and short plantar ligaments, and the plantar fasia. The transverse arch forms an arch from medial to lateral and consists of the navicular, cuneiforms, cuboid, and metatarsals and is supported by the tibialis anterior and posterior, peroneus longus, and the plantar fascia. The transverse arch is divided into the tarsal, posterior, and anterior metatarsal arches.

Arndt-Schultz principle: The amount of energy absorbed must be sufficient to stimulate the absorbing tissues or no reaction will occur.

arteriosclerosis: A disease in which there is progressive thickening and hardening of the walls of the arteries.

artery: A large blood vessel that carries oxygen-rich blood from the heart to the rest of the body.

arthokinematics: The study of joint movements.

arthralgia: Pain in a joint, not an inflammatory condition.

arthritis: Pain and stiffness characterized by inflammation of a joint.

arthroplasty: The replacement of a joint or joint surfaces to restore the integrity and function of the joint.

arthroscopy: A surgical procedure performed through an endoscope.

arthrosis: Degenerative disorder of a joint.

articulate: Referring to an articulation, a joint.

articulation: A joint, a place where two or more bones are joined in such a way as to allow motion; *see also* uniarticulate, biarticulate, and multiarticulate.

artificial respiration: The act of providing ventilation for a person who has stopped breathing.

ascorbic acid: Vitamin C.

aseptic: Relating to a state of sterility, the absence of pathogenic organisms.

asphyxia: Suffocation; a situation in which an individual is unable to obtain adequate oxygen.

aspiration: The inspiration of fluid or foreign bodies into the lungs, such as with vomitus.

assumption of risk: A written statement signed by an athlete or his or her legal guardians stating that they are aware of the dangers inherent in participation of the particular sport and voluntarily accept the risk.

asthma: Also known as reactive airway disease; a narrowing of the airway due to swelling, spasm, or inflammation of the submucosa.

astigmatism: A condition of the eye in which the cornea is not exactly spherical; can often be corrected with lenses.

asymmetrical: Not the same, as in comparing one body area to its counterpart; the opposite of symmetrical.

asystole: The cessation of heartbeats.

ataxia: Jerky, uncoordinated movements of the limbs; an inability to move in a smooth coordinated fashion.

Ath: Abbreviation for "athlete."

atheroma: Atherosclerosis; a narrowing of the blood vessels caused by fatty deposits on the inner walls.

athlete's foot: *See* tinea pedis.

atrial fibrillation: An irregular heartbeat in which the atria beat "out of sync" and are ineffective in circulating blood.

atrium (atria-plural): The upper chambers of the heart.

atrophy: A wasting away of tissue; often used to describe loss of muscle tone.

attenuation: Loss of radiant energy due to reflection, refraction, or absorption; a decrease in intensity due to absorption into deeper tissues.

auditory nerve: *See* vestibulocochlear nerve.

auricle: External ear.

auricular hematoma: An inflammation of the external ear caused by repeated friction; common in the sport of wrestling.

auscultation: Listening to body sounds, usually with a stethoscope.

autism: Also known as Kanner's syndrome; self-absorption to the point of loss of reality characterized by repetitive and limited actions.

autogenic inhibition: A reflex activation of the antagonist and relaxation of the agonist caused by a sudden stretch.

autograft: A tissue or organ transferred from one part of a patient's body to another.

autoimmune disease: A disorder of the body in which the immune system is unable to distinguish between foreign material and that of itself and thus attacks its own otherwise healthy tissues.

automatic external defibrillator: An electric device designed to apply a "shock" to the heart with the intent of returning the fibrillating heart to normal sinus rhythm.

autonomic nervous system: The nervous system responsible for involuntary functions.

avascular: Lack of blood supply.

avascular necrosis: Death of a tissue due to lack of blood supply.

average current: The amount of current applied over a given time.

avulsion: A tear in which part of the structure is completely torn away.

axial skeleton: The skull, thorax, and spine.

axilla: Pertaining to the space inferior to the shoulder joint; under the arm; armpit.

axillary nerve: A branch of the brachial plexus; it is responsible for supplying the teres minor and deltoid muscles.

axonotmesis: Axonal compression injury in which the endoneural sheath remains intact and thus regeneration could occur.

B

Babinski's reflex/sign: A test for upper motor neuron lesion. The test is performed by running a blunt object on the plantar aspect of the foot starting at the calcaneus and moving upward in an arc toward the great toe. In the adult, a positive test is indicated by extension of the great toe and splaying of the lateral toes. This response is opposite in the infant.

bacitracin: An antibacterial ointment.

bacteriostatic: Halting the growth of bacteria.

bacterium: A small unicellular microorganism that multiplies asexually through cell division.

bacteriuria: Bacteria in the urine indicating infection of the bladder or kidneys.

Baker's cyst: A synovial fluid swelling in the popliteal space first reported in 1877 by William Morrant Baker, MD (1839-1896).

balance: A state of equilibrium; a constant state of motion in which attempts are made to keep the center of gravity well within the base of support; ability to maintain posture either statically or dynamically.

ballistic stretching: A dynamic stretch.

bandage: A piece of cloth, gauze, or other material used to hold a dressing in place, or to immobilize an injured body part.

Bankart's lesion: An avulsion of the anterior glenoid fossa caused by anterior dislocation.

barbiturates: A group of drugs from barbituric acid that depress activity of the central nervous system; most are used as sleeping pills; a strong dependence is developed and barbituates can be fatal when taken with alcohol.

barium enema: An enema used during an x-ray assessment of the large intestine and rectum to check for disease.

baroreceptors: A nerve ending responsible for sensing changes in pressure.

baroreflex: A reflex triggered by baroreceptors in an attempt to maintain pressure.

Barton's fracture: A fracture/dislocation of the distal radius.

basal cell carcinoma: Skin cancer found most commonly on the face, neck, and arms; caused by excessive exposure to sunlight.

basal metabolic rate: The rate at which energy is consumed at absolute rest.

base of support: The surface area that is in contact with an external surface.

baseline: A starting point that serves as a basis for comparison.

basilar artery: Artery at the base of the brain. It later splits to form the two posterior cerebral arteries.

BCG vaccine: The vaccine for tuberculosis.

beam nonuniformity ration (BNR): The ratio of peak intensity to average intensity across an ultrasound head. A measure of the quality of the sound head. The closer the number is to one, the more even the beam.

beat: A waveform created by the combining of two waves from different circuits.

Becker's muscular dystrophy: A form of muscular dystrophy that starts later in life and advances more slowly; similar to Duschenne's; hereditary disease.

Bell's palsy: A unilateral paralysis of the face. The cause is unknown and usually resolves spontaneously. In some cases taste is affected and hearing becomes oversensitive.

Benazepril (Lotensin): An ACE inhibitor.

bends: *See* decompression sickness.

benign tumor: A tumor that is not cancerous.

Bennett's fracture: A fracture/dislocation of the first metacarpal at the carpometacarpal joint.

beta (β) endorphin: A hormone naturally occurring in the brain having pain control properties similar to opiates.

beta blocker: A pharmacologic agent that reduces heart rate and the strength of the beat; it is used to treat high blood pressure and other heart diseases.

beta carotene: A substance found in orange fruits and vegetables that is converted to vitamin A.

biarticulate: Referring to the crossing of two joints. Example, the extensor carpi radialis longus crosses and performs a function at the elbow joint as well as the wrist.

bifid: A division into lobes separated by a cleft.

bifocal: Glasses that are designed such that the upper portion of the lens restores distant vision while the lower portion of the lens restores near vision.

bilateral: Relating to both sides of the body.

bile: A substance produced by the liver responsible for the breakdown of fat and the removal of waste from the liver.

bile duct: The passageway from the liver to the gallbladder.

binging and purging: A characteristic behavior in individuals suffering from bulimia in which the individual eats to excess with gluttonous behavior and then either vomits or uses laxatives to rid him or herself of the food ingested.

biochemistry: The science of the chemistry involved in living organisms.

bioequivalent: A drug that has the same effect on the body as another drug.

biofeedback: A means of giving a patient immediate feedback about bodily functions which are usually unconscious.

biomechanics: The study involving the knowledge and methods of mechanics that are applied to a human body.

bipartate: Divided into two distinct parts.

biphasic current: A pulse that deviates from the iso-electric line first in one direction, then crosses the line and deviates in the other direction; *see also* alternating current; contrast to monophasic.

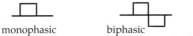

monophasic   biphasic

example of square monophasic and square biphasic waveforms.

bipolar arrangement: An electrical stimulation pad placement that uses two active electrodes (pads) of equal size.

bipolar cells: A neuron that has two processes off the cell body.

bladder: Internal organ responsible for storage of urine.

blood borne pathogen: Infectious disease carried in the blood.

blood doping: A technique used by athletes to increase the oxygen-carrying ability of the blood by giving a blood transfusion (just before an event) of one's own blood that was previously withdrawn.

blood poisoning: *See* septicemia.

blood pressure (BP): Pressure created by the blood on the walls of the arteries. The normal average BP for an adult is a systolic pressure of 120 and diastolic pressure of 80 (120/80).

blow-out fracture: A fracture of the floor of the eye's orbit produced by a blow to the globe of the eye.

body composition: A measure of the ratio of body fat to lean body weight.

boil: An inflammation of the skin containing pus caused by staphylococcus bacteria which enters through a hair follicle or skin wound. *See also* furuncle.

bone marrow: The yellow fatty (or red at birth) tissue within the central medullary cavity of bone responsible for producing blood cells.

bone marrow transplant: A surgical procedure in which bone marrow is removed from a healthy area within the patient's body or from a donor and transplanted to a diseased area.

bone spur: An abnormal bony outgrowth in response to repeated trauma; a common site of bone spur formation is the calcaneus at the plantar fascia attachment.

Borg scale: A rating of perceived exertion.

Borg Scale of Perceived Exertion	
Numeric Rating of Exertion	*Verbal Description of Exertion*
6	None
7	Very, very light
8	
9	Very light
10	
11	Fairly light
12	
13	Somewhat hard
14	
15	Hard
16	
17	Very hard
18	
19	Very, very hard
20	

botulism: A type of food poisoning which occurs from ingestion of the neurotoxin *clostridium botulinum*, commonly occurring in improperly canned food.

bounce home test: A special test of the knee for meniscal injury. *See* Special Tests—Knee (Appendix 16).

boutonnière deformity: An injury to the extensor hood of the phalanges that causes flexion of the proximal interphalangeal and extension of the distal interphalangeal.

boxer's fracture: A fracture of the neck of a metacarpal (usually the fifth) with a volar displacement of the head of the metacarpal.

bowstring test: A special test for sciatic nerve involvement. *See* Special Tests—Spine (Appendix 16).

brachial plexus: A network of nerves made up of nerve roots (C4) C5-T1 that blend and divide to form a network and terminate as the peripheral nerves that supply the arm (axillary, musculocutaneous, median, ulnar, and radial nerves).

brachio: Arm.

brachy: Short.

bradycardia: An abnormally slow heart rate (less than 60 beats per minute).

bradykinin: A polypeptide hormone composed of a chain of nine amino acid residues formed during the inflammatory process causing vasodilation; responsible in part for the sensation of pain.

break test: A common method of assessing resistive range of motion. The patient is placed in mid range and the examiner attempts to "break" the contraction of the patient.

bronchitis: Inflammation of the mucous membranes of the bronchials.

bronchoconstrictor: A substance that causes the bronchial tubes to constrict or become smaller in diameter.

bronchodilator: A pharmacologic agent that dilates or increases the diameter of the bronchial tubes to improve breathing.

bronchospasm: A constriction of narrowing of the airway as a result of muscle contraction or inflammation; may be exercised induced (EIA-exercise-induced asthma), allergen induced, or caused by infection or other lung disease.

Brudzinski's sign: A variation of the straight leg raise in which neck flexion is combined with a straight leg raise. A positive sign of pain in the lumbar region or legs indicates nerve involvement.

bruise: *See* contusion.

bruxism: An involuntary action of grinding the teeth.

buccal: Referring to the cheek or mouth.

bulimia: A disorder in which the patient binges (ie, eats large amounts of food) and then purges the food by vomiting or using laxatives.

bunion: Localized inflammation and calcification of the first metatarsophalangeal joint either dorsal or medial; often associated with hallux valgus.

Bunnel-Littler test: A special test of the proximal interphalangeal joint to determine cause of tightness. *See* Special Tests—Hand/Wrist (Appendix 16).

burner: *See* neurapraxia.

bursa: A closed sac lined with synovial membrane containing fluid; acts as a cushion and lubricant and is found in areas subjected to friction.

bursitis: Inflammation of the bursa.

bursts: A series of electrical pulses delivered in packets or beats.

bypass: A shunt; a surgical technique in which a new path is created from which the flow of blood can "bypass" a blockage.

C

C fiber: An afferent neuron responsible for carrying temperature and noxious stimuli; responsible for "slow pain."

CAAHEP: *See* Commission of Accreditation of Allied Health Education Programs.

calcific tendonitis: Deposits of calcium in a tendon following chronic tendonitis.

calcification: The process in which calcium salts are deposited in the tissue.

calcium: Mineral that aids in nerve transmission, muscle contraction, blood clotting, heart functioning, and also works with enzymes.

callus: A thickening of the skin caused by repeated friction; new bone formation.

calor: Heat.

calorie: A unit of heat; the unit of measure for the amount of energy contained in food; the amount of heat required to raise 1 kg of water 1°C.

cancer: A term for malignant neoplasm.

candidiasis: An infection or disease caused by *Candida albicans*; occurs commonly in the vagina, and less commonly in the mouth, or on the penis.

capacitance: The ability to store and separate an electric charge; the elasticity of a tissue.

capsular pattern: An abnormal movement pattern characteristic of each joint when there is capsular involvement.

captopril (Capoten): An ACE inhibitor.

carbohydrate: One of a group of compounds (mainly sugar and starch), made up of carbon, hydrogen, and oxygen; a main source of energy for the body that is eventually broken down to a simple sugar. Excess carbohydrate is stored in muscles and the liver as glycogen.

carbon dioxide: A colorless gas present in small amounts in the atmosphere and formed during metabolism; it is carried through the blood to the lungs where it is exhaled.

carcinogen: Any cancer-causing substance.

carcinoma: A cancer that occurs on epithelial tissue.

cardiac arrest: The sudden cessation of effective pumping action of the heart due to fibrillation or asystole.

cardinal planes: Three imaginary perpendicular reference planes that divide the body into left and right, front and back, and upper and lower halves.

cardiomyopathy: A chronic disease of the heart muscle.

cardiopulmonary resuscitation (CPR): The administration of external cardiac compressions and artificial respiration to restore circulation.

cardiovascular system: The system responsible for circulating blood throughout the body including the heart and blood vessels.

carotene: An orange pigment (lipochrome) present in colored plants such as carrots; they include the precursor to the essential nutrient vitamin A.

carotid arteries: The two main arteries that carry blood to the head and neck (they further divide into the external and internal carotid arteries bilaterally).

carpal tunnel syndrome: One of the most common nerve entrapment syndromes. The median nerve becomes entrapped under the transverse carpal ligament. Characterized by pain and paresthesia in the median nerve distribution of the hand. Atrophy of the thenar eminence can occur.

carpals: Small bones of the hand (proximal row from lateral to medial: scaphoid, lunate, triquetrum, pisiform) (distal row from lateral to medial: trapezium, trapezoid, capitate, hamate).

cartilage: An avascular connective tissue including hyaline, elastic, and fibrocartilage commonly found on bone ends, walls of the thorax, and tubular structures such as the ear canal and the airway. Most of the fetal skeleton is composed of cartilage and is later replaced by bone.

cast: A method of immobilization which often employs a plaster of paris or fiberglass shell.

catalysis: An increase in the rate of a chemical reaction induced by a catalyst.

catalyst: An enzyme that stimulates a chemical reaction to occur where it normally would be impossible, such as allowing a chemical reaction to occur at a temperature lower than it could usually occur.

cataract: Opacity or loss of transparency of the lens of the eye causing blurred vision.

catheter: A hollow tube-like device used to allow the passage of fluid.

catheterization: The insertion of a catheter or tube to permit influx or withdrawal of fluids.

cathode: The negative electrode.

cauda equina: The distal end of the spinal cord that forms the roots of the upper sacral nerves at the L1 level; resembles a "horse's tail."

cauda equina syndrome: Injury to the cauda equina often from disk lesion characterized by bilateral leg pain, diminished deep tendon reflexes, and bowel or bladder dysfunction. The patient with suspected cauda equina syndrome should be referred immediately to a physician.

caudal: Toward the tail.

cauliflower ear: *See* auricular hematoma.

cauterization: The use of a cautery, a device that burns tissue with cryo-, thermo-, or electrotherapy to stop bleeding.

cavitation: Gaseous bubbles formed by the mechanical effect of therapeutic ultrasound.

cecum: The proximal end of the large intestine.

cell: The smallest living structure capable of independence; composed of a nucleus and a cell membrane made up of lipids and proteins capable of reproducing itself.

cellulitis: Inflammation of cellular connective tissue caused by bacterial infection often requiring the use of antibiotics.

center of balance: The point in the center between the feet or in the middle of the foot (in a single limb stance) in which 25% of the body weight falls in each of four quadrants measured two-dimensionally.

center of gravity: The central point about which the mass of an object is equally distributed.

center of pressure: Vertical ground reaction forces representing the center of the deviations measured three-dimensionally.

central biasing: Also known as descending inhibition; a theory of pain control in which pain is diminished through efferent impulses having left the higher centers to "block the gate" of pain transmission.

central nervous system: The part of the nervous system consisting of the brain and spinal cord.

centrifugal force: The force exerted radially outward on a body that is rotating about an axis.

centripetal force: The force exerted radially inward that is causing a body to travel in a circular path.

cephalad: Meaning toward the head.

cerebellum: The largest part of the posterior brain; responsible for muscle tone, balance, and smooth coordinated movement, although not responsible for the initiation of voluntary motions.

cerebral palsy: A disorder commonly occurring before birth in which damage to the brain occurs causing weakness, uncoordinated movement of the limbs, and often affecting speech; spastic cerebral palsy is characterized by contractures which can progress to permanent deformity; uncontrolled writhing movements, called athetosis, are also common; causes include lack of oxygen, viral infection, and meningitis.

cerebrospinal fluid (CSF): A clear, watery fluid found in the subarachnoid space surrounding the brain and spinal column made up of glucose, salts, enzymes, and white blood cells.

cerebrovascular disease: Illness affecting the arteries that supply the brain; can lead to the formation of a blockage, resulting in a cerebrovascular accident, or stroke.

cerumen: Soft, waxy, brown secretion of the external auditory meatus.

cervix: A neck-like structure at the distal end of the uterus.

cesarean section: A surgical procedure to remove the fetus from the womb through the abdominal wall; used when the health of the infant and/or mother would be at risk during natural childbirth.

continuing education units (CEU): NATABOC Athletic trainers are required to complete 80 CEUs every 3 years.

chafing: A superficial skin wound caused by friction from skin rubbing skin.

chancre: A painless sore that occurs on the lips, eyelids, or genitals; a common sign of the sexually transmitted disease syphilis.

Charcot's syndrome: A disease of the spinal cord affecting one or more joints and ultimately resulting in a flail joint.

chemoreceptors: Afferent receptors sensitive to chemical changes.

chemotherapy: The use of chemical substances to treat infectious diseases and cancer.

Cheyne-Stokes breathing: An abnormal pattern of breathing in which the rate increases and decreases over a 1 minute period.

chi square (c^2): A nonparametric statistical technique used to determine the significance between frequencies of nominal data.

chickenpox: Varicella, a highly contagious disease transmitted by airborne herpes virus characterized by fever and itchy red pimples; occurs most commonly during childhood.

cholecyst: The gallbladder.

cholecystectomy: The surgical removal of the gallbladder.

cholera: An acute epidemic disease caused by *vibrio cholerae*, causing severe diarrhea leading to dehydration, and possibly death.

cholesterol: A fatty substance in blood and other tissues; important precursor of steroid hormones and bile salts; elevated levels associated with atheroma.

cholinergic: Nerve fibers that release acetylcholine as a neurotransmitter.

chondral: Cartilage.

chondral fracture: A fracture that also involves the articular cartilage of a joint.

chondritis: Inflammation of cartilage.

chondroma: A benign tumor in the cartilage.

chondromalacia: A degenerative condition is which there is a wearing away of the cartilage; on the posterior surface of the patella in chondromalacia patella.

chondrosarcoma: A malignant tumor that develops on the surface of a bone in the cartilage.

chronaxie: The phase duration required to cause an action potential when intensity is two times the rheobase.

chronic: Gradual onset; a disease or injury with a long duration.

cilia: Eyelash; a small, hair-like, motile structure found on the outside of some cells.

ciliary muscle: The muscle that controls the curvature of the lens of the eye.

CINAHL (Cumulative Index to Nursing and Allied Health Literature): An online resource for nursing and allied health professionals covering nursing, biomedicine, health sciences librarianship, consumer health, and 17 allied health disciplines. CINAHL indexes over 1200 nursing journals and other publications. It dates back to 1982.

circadian rhythm: The biological time clock.

circumduction: A circular movement made by a limb such as that made when one swings ones arms in a circle;

the combined motions of flexion, extension, abduction, adduction.

cirrhosis of the liver: A progressive disease of the liver in which there is a gradual loss of liver function due to cell damage; there are many causes including long-term alcoholism.

Clancy test: A special test of the shoulder used to test for a slap lesion. *See* Special Test—Shoulder (Appendix 16).

Clark's sign test: Also called patellar crunch or grind; a special test for chondromalacia of the patella performed by stabilizing the patella at the superior pole and asking the patient to contract the quadriceps. A positive test is indicated by pain.

claudication: Ischemia most commonly of the triceps surae; a cramping pain in one or both legs while walking, which can cause limping.

claustrophobia: A fear of being in confined or crowded spaces.

clavicle: The horizontal s-shaped bone that runs from the sternum to the acromion process of the scapula; commonly referred to as the collarbone.

claw toes: Characteristic extension of the MTP joints and flexion of the IP joints.

clawfoot: *See* pes cavus.

cleft lip: Harelip; a cleft palate that extends the entire palate and to the lip.

cleft palate: A fissure in the palate resulting from a birth defect in which the two sides of the palate fail to fuse together; can also occur with other birth defects such as cleft lip and partial deafness.

clinical instructor educator (CIE): A certified athletic trainer who has successfully completed the CIE training workshop and will train the approved clinical instructors for his or her academic program.

clinical trial: A research study involving a new drug or treatment.

clonus: Rhythmical limb movements such as those seen during a convulsive episode.

closed basket weave: Gibney technique; a taping procedure for ankle mediolateral instability.

closed (kinetic) chain: Referring to motion that takes place in which the proximal segments rotate about the fixed distal segment.

closed fracture: A bone break that does not break the skin.

closed packed position: A joint position when the bone ends are most congruent.

closed reduction: The act of repositioning a displaced joint or bone without the need for surgery.

clubfoot: *See* talipes equinovarus.

coccyx: The distal bones of the spine which include four small fused bones forming a triangular shape at the base of the spine.

cochlea: The spiraled organ in the inner ear that picks up vibrations and transforms them into electrical signals that in turn are sent to the brain and interpreted as sound.

co-contraction: A muscular contraction in which both agonist and antagonist muscles contract simultaneously.

Codman's exercise: Pendulum exercises; passive range of motion exercises for the shoulder performed by the patient.

coefficient of friction: The ratio of the friction force to the perpendicular (normal) force pushing the two objects together.

colic: Severe waves of pain in the abdomen or urinary tract (in renal colic-kidney stones) often caused by a stone or intestinal infection.

colitis: Inflammation of the colon leading to abdominal pain, fever, and bloody diarrhea.

collateral: Accompanying, side by side; often used pertaining to the lateral ligaments on either side of the knee including the medial (tibial) collateral and the lateral (fibular) collateral ligament.

Colles' wrist fracture: A fracture of the distal radius in which there is a backward displacement below the fracture site.

colon: The distal end of the large intestine, between the cecum and the rectum.

colonectomy: The complete or partial removal of the colon (large intestine).

colonoscopy: Visual examination of the colon using a long, flexible fiberoptic tube.

colostomy: A surgical procedure in which a stoma is formed by attaching the colon to the abdomen and thus making a new opening for feces to be excreted into a bag worn on the abdomen; see also ileostomy.

coma: A state of unconsciousness in which the individual cannot be aroused or can be aroused only minimally; the Glasgow coma scale is a means of "grading" the condition and takes into account whether the individual responds to verbal or painful stimuli.

comminuted fracture: A fracture in which there are many small pieces.

Commission of Accreditation of Allied Health Education Programs (CAAHEP): The accrediting body for several allied health professions, including athletic training education programs.

communicable disease: A disease that can be spread from one individual to another.

compartment syndrome: A condition in which inflammation causes increased pressure in a compartment and thus increased pressure on the nerves and blood supply that are contained in the compartment. Occurs commonly in the compartments of the lower leg, especially the anterior compartment. Onset of compartment syndrome can be acute or chronic.

compliance: The extent to which the patient adheres to medical advice.

compound fracture: An open fracture; a fracture in which the bone ends protrude through the skin.

compression fracture: A fracture in which a bone is broken due to compressive forces.

compression test: Special test of the cervical spine for nerve root compression. *See* Special Tests—Spine (Appendix 16).

computed tomography scanning: CT, CAT scan; a radiological technique for producing cross-sectional images of the body that are then analyzed with a computer.

concave: A surface that is curved inward.

concave-convex rule: In joint mobilization, the rule related to movement of a concave bone on a convex bone describing accessory motion that is in the same direction as the physiological motion. *See also* convex-concave rule.

concentric contraction: A muscular contraction in which the muscle is shortening.

concussion: An injury to the brain caused by a blow to the head in which there are disturbances in the electrical activity in the brain; symptoms include headache, nausea, loss of consciousness, memory loss, and other neuropsychological impairment. Common grading systems and return to play criteria can be found in Appendix 8.

conduction: A method of heat transfer through direct contact with an object of a different temperature.

confidence interval: A pair of numbers on either end of a range from a sample that has a particular probability of including the population parameters.

congenital: Describing that which was present at the time of birth.

congestive heart failure: A condition in which the heart is ineffective at circulating blood and results in fluid accumulation and congestion of the lungs.

conjunctiva: The clear membrane that covers the front of the eye and lines the eyelids.

conjunctivitis: Also known as pink eye; inflammation of the conjunctiva caused by allergy, chemical reaction, or virus, in which case it will quickly spread to the other eye.

connective tissue: Strong fibrous tissue that connects and supports body structures including tendon, ligaments, cartilage, bone, adipose tissue, and elastic structures.

constipation: A condition in which there are incomplete or infrequent bowel movements and feces are dry and hard.

continuous passive motion machine (CPMM): A device used to provide passive movement of a joint; usually used following surgery to reduce loss of motion.

contracture: Muscle shortening due to muscle spasm or fibrosis.

contraindication: A treatment not recommended or inadvisable due to the current condition.

contralateral: Denoting the opposite side.

contrecoup injury: Lesion within the skull opposite to the side in which the blow occurred.

contusion: Internal damage to the tissue as a result of a blunt trauma resulting in discoloration.

convection: A method of heat transfer in which heat is transferred indirectly through medium such as air or liquid.

convex: A surface that is curved outward; *see also* convex-concave rule.

convex-concave rule: In joint mobilization, the rule related to movement of a convex bone on a concave bone describing accessory motion that is in the direction opposite the physiological motion. *See also* concave-convex rule.

convulsions: Waves of involuntary muscular contractions and relaxations.

core stability: A fine line between mobility and stability, it is functional stability of the trunk with appropriate biomechanical alignment between the pelvis and shoulder girdle and efficient, coordinated neuromuscular recruitment of the trunk.

corn: A thickened callus that forms over a bony prominence, commonly in the toes.

cornea: Continuous with the conjunctiva, it is the clear, anterior one-sixth of the eye, serving as the main refractory structure of the eye focusing light on the retina.

coronal plane: Also known as frontal plane; divides the body into dorsal and ventral or anterior and posterior parts. Motions that take place in this plane include abduction/adduction, radial/ulnar deviation, and lateral flexion of the trunk and head.

corticosteroids: Any steroid synthesized by the adrenal cortex; synthetic corticosteroids are used for the powerful anti-inflammatory effect created by suppression of the immune system.

coryza: Inflammation of the mucous membrane of the nasal airway caused by the common cold or allergies.

cosine law: Electromagnetic radiations travel in a straight line, therefore the ideal position is at a right angle to the target tissue.

costo: Denoting the ribs.

costochondral: The junction of the ribs and the cartilage between the ribs and the sternum.

costoclavicular: The articulation of the ribs and clavicle.

costoclavicular syndrome test: A special test of the shoulder to assess thoracic outlet syndrome. *See* Special Tests—Shoulder (Appendix 16).

counterirritant: An agent that creates a mild irritation and acts as an analgesic. Examples include heat, cold, and superficial analgesics.

coupling medium: A substance used to reduce impedance and facilitate conductivity.

coxa: Hip.

coxa plana: A degenerative disease of the capital femoral epiphysis. *See also* Legg-Calvé-Perthes disease.

coxa valgus: A condition in which the angle between the axis of the femoral neck and the long axis of the femoral shaft is greater than 135 degrees.

coxa vara: A condition in which the angle between the axis of the femoral neck and the long axis of the femoral shaft is less than 135 degrees.

coxalgia: Hip pain.

creatine: A substance that combines with phosphate to form creatine phosphate (phosphocreatine) a high-energy phosphate released during anaerobic muscular activity. Recently taken as a supplement. Side effects and effects of long-term use are not fully understood.

creatinine: A urinary waste product of phosphocreatine metabolism produced by the kidneys. The normal creatinine level is 1.2 mg/dL.

crepitation: Fine crackling sensation such as that felt when palpating over a fracture site.

crepitus: A grating sensation in a joint or tendon due to swelling or degenerative changes.

criterion referenced tests: Tests which have a predetermined standard of performance.

Crohn's disease: Ulcerative colitis; inflammatory disease affecting the distal end of the ileum in which there is thickening and ulcerations. Treatment includes antibiotics, immunosuppressive drugs, and in some cases removal of the affected part of the intestine.

cross-arm adduction test: *See* cross-over impingement test.

cross-over impingement test: A special test of the shoulder to assess impingement. *See* Special Tests—Shoulder (Appendix 16).

crural index: The ratio of upper leg length to leg length.

cryokinetics: Application of cold prior to or simultaneous to an exercise regime.

cryotherapy: Treatment involving the use of cold and ice.

CT scanning: *See* computed tomography scanning.

cubital tunnel: A tunnel formed by the ulna, ulnar collateral ligament, and the flexor carpi ulnaris muscle through which the ulnar nerve passes.

cubital tunnel syndrome: Compression of the ulnar nerve as it passes through the cubital tunnel.

culture: The propagation of cells or microorganisms in a laboratory setting.

current density: Amount of electrical current per given area.

curvilinear: The path of movement along a curved line.

cyanosis: A bluish discoloration of the skin beginning around the lips, caused by reduced oxygen levels.

cyclist's knee: *See* iliotibial band friction syndrome; also known as runner's knee.

cyst: Abnormal closed sac filled with fluid and lined with epithelial tissue.

cystectomy: Surgical removal of the bladder; a length of the small intestine can be used to form a "new bladder," or in some cases a urostomy is necessary.

cystic fibrosis: A genetic disorder affecting the exocrine glands resulting in production of a thick mucous which can obstruct the lungs, pancreas, or intestinal glands; infection is common; treatment is aimed at reducing bronchial stress and preventing infection.

cystoscopy: Examination of the bladder and urethra using cystescope.

Daily Adjustable Progressive Resistance Exercise (DAPRE): Developed by Ken Knight, this is a protocol involving of increased resistance exercise 6 days per week in which the following procedure is followed: the first set consists of 10 repetitions at 50%, followed by the second set consisting of 6 repetitions at 75%, followed by the third set consisting of as many repetitions as possible at 100%, followed by the fourth set of as many as possible adjusted from the first set as described next. The fourth set is adjusted based on the number of repetitions performed in the third as follows: 0 to 2 repetitions, decrease weight and redo set; 3 to 4 repetitions, decrease by 5 pounds; 5 to 7 repetitions, use the same weight; 8 to 12 repetitions, increase by 5 to 10 pounds; 13+ repetitions, increase 10 to 15 pounds.

de Quervain's disease: Tenosynovitis of the extensor pollicus brevis and abductor pollicus longus caused by repetitive motions.

deafferentation: A loss or reduction of afferent input.

debridement: The removal of foreign material and dead tissue from an open wound.

decay: Tissue death.

deceleration: Decrease in velocity per unit of time (meters per second per second—m/s^2). For example, $-1\ m/s^2$ means that velocity is decreased by 1 m/s every second.

decerebrate (rigidity): Abnormal posture indicating brain stem injury, extension and adduction of the upper extremity joints and extension, internal rotation and plantar flexion in the lower extremity.

decompression sickness: "The bends"; a common injury in scuba diving caused by ascending too quickly; gas bubbles are formed in the body's tissues.

deconditioning: A period in which an athlete loses his or her fitness level.

decorticate (rigidity): Abnormal posture indicating injury above the brainstem, flexion, and adduction of the upper extremity joints, extension, internal rotation, and plantar flexion in the lower extremity.

deep tendon reflex: An involuntary muscular contraction controlled by the reflex arc and caused by a sudden stretch imposed on a tendon.

deep-vein thrombophlebitis: A thrombosis associated with inflammation of a vein wall.

deep-vein thrombosis: A blood clot commonly occurring in the veins of lower leg, causing pain.

defecation: The act of moving the bowels.

defibrillation: The use of an electric shock in an attempt to re-synchronize the defibrillating heart.

deficit: A decrease in functional capacity as when compared bilaterally or to the norm.

degenerative arthritis: *See* osteoarthritis.

degrees: A unit of measure for range of motion in which a complete circle is divided into 360 equal parts; a unit of measure for temperature.

degrees of freedom: The number of variables that are free to vary when restrictions are set.

dehydration: A condition in which there is a severe loss of fluid (water) from the body.

dementia: Alzheimer's disease is the most commonly known form of dementia; a gradual decline in mental ability.

dendrite: A branching process of a neuron that conducts impulses toward the soma (cell body).

density: Mass or weight per unit volume.

dental caries: Cavities or tooth decay.

dependent variable: Dependent measure; in research, it is the variable that is measured.

depolarization: The act of neutralizing a cell membrane's resting potential.

depression: A lowering or downward movement.

dermabrasion: A procedure in which the surface of skin is removed through abrasion, commonly with a sanding device; a common treatment for scarring or the removal of tattoos.

dermatitis: Inflammation of the skin.

dermatome: A sensory area of the skin supplied by a particular nerve root.

dermis: The deep layer of skin.

descriptive statistics: The statistics used to describe a set of data.

deviate: To vary from the norm.

deviated septum: Displacement of the ethmoid and/or vomar bones causing disruption of continuity of the nasal septum.

deviation score: The difference of a score from the mean.

dextrose: Glucose.

diabetes insipidus: A rare metabolic condition characterized by increased urine production treated with the hormone vasopressin.

diabetes mellitus: A common form of diabetes in which glucose is not oxidized due to the lack of insulin production from the pancreas. Control is maintained by dietary intake and the use of insulin.

diagnosis: A process of disease identification through its signs and symptoms.

dialysis: A process in which blood is removed from an artery and enters a dialyzer (filtering machine); the blood is filtered and returns through a vein. This procedure is used to treat kidney failure to remove waste products, maintain acid-base balance, and remove excess fluid from the body.

diapedesis: Emigration; the passage of blood cells through the intact capillary wall.

diaphragm: A large muscle found between the abdomen and chest cavity responsible for breathing. When the diaphragm contracts, pressure in the chest increases and forces air in the airway into the lungs. When the diaphragm relaxes, air is expelled through the airway. Also, a thin, latex, dome-shaped apparatus used as a method of contraception.

diaphysis: The shaft of a long bone.

diarthrodial: A ball and socket type of joint.

diastole: The relaxation period of the heart between two contractions at which time the heart chamber fills with blood.

diastolic pressure: The blood pressure measured when the heart is in diastole (relaxation phase in which the ventricle fills with blood); the normal systolic pressure in an adult is 120 mmHg, normal diastolic pressure in an adult is 80 mmHg, recorded as 120/80 mmHg.

diathermy: A deep heating modality from the electromagnetic spectrum that uses high frequency electromagnetic energy. Shortwave diathermy has wavelengths ranging from 11 to 22 m and operates at a frequency of approximately 13 to 27 MHz; microwave diathermy has wavelengths ranging from 12 to 70 cm and operates at a frequency of approximately 430 to 2,450 MHz.

differential diagnosis: A process of diagnosing an injury or illness which shares common signs and symptoms with other conditions, and thus must be ruled out.

diplegia: Bilateral paralysis, often more severe in the legs.

diplopia: Double vision.

direct current: An electrical current that does not alternate polarity; does not cross the isoelectric line.

direct service: Treatment or other services provided directly to one or more patients by a practitioner.

disk injury: Herniated disk; bulging disk; injury to the annulus fibrosis (outer covering) of the vertebral disk in which a portion of disk material protrudes and places pressure on a nerve root, causing numbness, tingling, weakness, impaired deep tendon reflexes, and most commonly pain along the nerve distribution. The severity of injury depends on the amount of pressure applied and by the disk material as well as secondary swelling. Protrusion, prolapse, extrusion, and sequestration are common disk injuries.

dislocation: A third-degree sprain in which two or more bones are displaced at the joint. A partial, incomplete, or an immediate and spontaneous relocation is referred to as a subluxation.

dispersive electrode: A large "not active" electrode used to complete the electrical circuit. Due to its size, current density is small and thus the dispersive electrode is not an "active" electrode. The use of a dispersive pad constitutes a monopolar pad placement.

distal: Further away from the point of origin.

distention: Stretching as in the bladder or stomach; swelling, enlargement.

distraction: To pull apart; a special test in which a joint is distracted (pulled apart) causing a reduction of symptoms.

diuretic: A pharmacologic agent designed to increase the amount of water in the urine thereby removing excess water from the body; commonly used to treat fluid retention and hypertension.

diverticula: Small sacs on the inner lining of the intestine.

diverticulitis: Inflammation of diverticula.

deoxyribonucleic acid (DNA): the genetic make-up of all living organisms.

domain: A specific performance area. The 12 domains in athletic training education include "risk management and injury prevention," "pathology of injuries and illnesses," "assessment and evaluation," "acute care of injuries and illnesses," "pharmacology," "therapeutic modalities," "therapeutic exercise," "general medical conditions," "nutritional aspects," "psychosocial intervention and referral," "health care administration," and "professional development and responsibility."

dominant gene: A powerful gene in that whenever it is present, it always produces its effect.

don: To put on clothing.

dorsal: Pertaining to the back; dorsum.

dorsiflexion: Flexion of the foot toward the shin; to bring the "toes up."

Down syndrome: Trisomy 21, a genetic disorder in which there are three number 21 chromosomes, causing moderate to severe mental handicap and a characteristic appearance of slanted eyes, small ears, flat nose bridge, and short stature.

downward rotation: Movement of the scapula such that the glenoid fossa move downward.

dressing: A covering on a wound.

drop arm test: A special test of the shoulder for rotator cuff injury. *See* Special Tests—Shoulder (Appendix 16).

drop foot syndrome: A condition caused by weakness of the dorsiflexors in which the individual is unable to dorsiflex and thus unable to support the foot during the swing phase of the gait, therefore the foot "drops."

Duchenne's muscular dystrophy (MD): *See* muscular dystrophy.

Dupuytren's contracture: An abnormal fusion of the flexor tendon to the skin of the third and fourth fingers, causing a flexion contracture.

dura: The thick, outermost covering of the brain and spinal cord.

duration: Length of time; in modalities it refers to treatment time; the measure of the length of time of an electromagnetic wave (ie, the phase duration of the pulse is 200 microseconds).

duty cycle: A relationship of the on time to the off time over a specified period. A treatment in which there is a 5 msec on time and 5 msec off time has a 50% duty cycle.

dynamic flexibility: The available range of motion during active (dynamic) motion; a type of flexibility exercise performed quickly, under dynamic/ballistic loads.

dynamic splint: A splint that is designed to provide continuous passive or active assisted stretch.

dynamometer: A device used to record muscular force.

dyspnea: Difficulty breathing.

E

eccentric contraction: A muscular contraction which takes place during muscular lengthening.

ecchymosis: Bruise, contusion, caused by the escape of blood into the tissues.

echocardiogram: An ultrasound image of the heart.

ectomorph: A somatotype (ie, body type) characterized by being tall and thin.

ectopic: Located in an abnormal position.

eczema: Inflammation of the skin characterized by itching and scales; cause is often unknown, can occur due to allergies.

edema: Accumulation of fluid in the body; in injury, caused by the effects of inflammation.

effective radiating area (ERA): The area of the sound head (ultrasound) which has been deemed to effectively deliver ultrasound. For example, an ultrasound head that measures 5 cm^2 may only have an ERA of 4.7 cm^2. In order to be considered in the ERA, 5% of the initial intensity must be measurable at a depth of 5 cm.

efferent: Conducting away from the center. In the case of nerves, conducting away from the brain, responsible for conducting impulses from the brain to the organs.

efficacy: The capability of having the desired effect.

effleurage: A type of therapeutic massage involving a rhythmical motion in one direction with the intent of increasing blood flow.

effusion: Excess blood or fluid in the tissues.

Ehlers-Danlos syndrome: A genetic disorder of connective tissue characterized by hypermobility of the joints, delicate skin that bruises easily, subcutaneous cysts, and visceral deformity.

elastic limit: Yield point; the point on a stress strain curve at which further stress will cause permanent deformation.

elastic modulus: The ratio of stress to strain (ie, the slope of the line).

elasticity: The ability to return to its original shape once tension is released.

elbow flexion test: A special test of the elbow to assess ulnar nerve entrapment. *See* Special Tests—Elbow (Appendix 16).

elective: Referring to a treatment or procedure that is not necessary and can be "elected" as a form of treatment by the patient; often not covered by medical insurance.

electrical impedance: Resistance, the opposition to electron flow.

electrocardiogram (ECG or EKG): An instrument that measures the electrical impulses of the heartbeat.

electroencephalography: A process of assessing brain activity by recording the brain's electrical impulses.

electrogoniometer: An electrical device used to measure range of motion.

electromagnetic field: Forms of energy emanating from an electrical source; an electrical field created by the lines of force between the two poles.

electromagnetic spectrum: A means of displaying the relationship between various forms of energy by placing them along a continuum arranged in order by wavelength, including cosmic and gamma rays, visible light, infrared modalities, and electrical stimulating modalities.

elevation: An upward movement of the scapula.

Ely's: A special test of the hip to assess hip flexion contracture, specifically the rectus femoris. *See* Special Tests—Hip (Appendix 16).

embolism: The blockage caused by an embolus.

embolus: Material in the blood, such as a blood clot, fat, air, bacteria, amniotic fluid, bone marrow, cholesterol, etc, that circulates in the blood from one place to another and becomes lodged.

embryo: An animal in the early stages of development; in humans it refers to the first 8 weeks following fertilization.

empty can test (supraspinatus test): A special test of the shoulder to assess the rotator cuff. *See* Special Tests—Shoulder (Appendix 16).

EMS: Abbreviation for "emergency medical services" or "electrical muscle stimulation." For this reason, NMES (neuromuscular electrical stimulation) is preferred.

end feel: The normal or abnormal sensation or resistance felt by the examiner at the end of a passive range of motion. *See* Appendix 15.

endemic: Describes a disease that tends to be present within a certain group of people.

endocrine gland: A hormone-secreting gland that secretes directly into the blood. The pituitary, thyroid, parathyroid, adrenal, ovaries, and testes are examples of endocrine glands.

endogenous: Arising from inside of the body.

endogenous opioids: A hormone naturally occurring in the brain having pain control properties similar to opiates.

endometriosis: The presence of endometrium in other areas of the pelvis causing severe pain lasting several days each month.

endometrium: The membrane lining the uterus.

endomorph: A somatotype (ie, body type) characterized by being short and overweight.

endorphin: One of a group of naturally occurring chemicals produced in the brain exhibiting strong pain relieving properties similar to that of opiates.

endoscope: A lighted instrument with an optical system used to transmit images from the inside of a body cavity.

endothelium: A thin layer of tissue cells that line the heart, blood, and lymphatic vessels.

endpoint: *See* end feel.

endurance: The ability to perform activity for an extended period of time without fatigue; the ability to bear pain, adversity, and stress.

energy: The capacity to perform work.

enkephalin: A protein neurotransmitter that inhibits the release of substance P, thereby blocking the transmission of noxious stimuli from first order to second order neurons.

enteritis: Inflammation of the small intestine.

enuresis: Bed wetting.

enzyme: a protein that speeds up biological reactions.

epicondylitis: Inflammation of the epicondyle at the origin of the wrist extensors (lateral epicondylitis) or wrist flexors (medial epicondylitis).

epidemic: A sudden outbreak of an illness that spreads rapidly.

epidemiology: The study of epidemic disease for the purpose of discovering its cause and preventing future cases.

epidermis: The outermost layer of skin.

epidural anesthesia: A procedure to block pain in which a pain-relieving pharmacologic agent is injected into the epidural space around the spinal cord to block sensation to the abdomen and lower extremities; this procedure is commonly used during childbirth or for lower extremity surgery.

epidural hematoma: Bleeding in the brain above the dura matter, usually arterial bleeding with rapid onset of symptoms. Compare to subdural hematoma.

epilepsy: A disorder of unknown cause affecting the nervous system in which there is abnormal electrical activity in the brain causing petit mal and grand mal seizures; epilepsy is controlled with anticonvulsant drugs such as dilantin.

epinephrine: Also known as adrenaline; a hormone secreted by the adrenal glands in response to stress or fear;

responsible for the "fight-or-flight" response in which there is an increase in heart rate, metabolism, and improved breathing.

epiphysis: The end of a long bone, separated from the diaphysis by the metaphysis to allow for bone growth which eventually fuses to the diaphysis.

epitaxis: Nosebleed.

epithelium: Tissue covering the external surface of the body and lining the hollow organs.

Epstein-Barr virus: A virus that causes mononucleosis; spread by mucous secretions.

equinus deformity: A congenital deformity of the foot in which there is a contracture of the plantar flexors of the foot; gait is marked by toe walking.

Erb palsy: A birth defect in which there is a lesion to the upper trunk of the brachial plexus or the nerve roots from C5-6 causing weakness or paralysis of the deltoid, biceps, brachialis, and brachioradialis.

ergonomics: The study of man in his work surroundings.

erysipelas: Fever and rash caused by streptococci bacteria.

erythema: Redness of the skin.

erythrocyte: Red blood cell.

erythroplakia: A precursor to cancer characterized by red patches in the mucous membranes of the mouth, throat, or larynx; tobacco users have increased risk.

esophageal spasm: A contraction of the smooth muscle of the esophagus that causes difficulty swallowing.

esophagus: The portion of the digestive tract connecting the throat to the stomach.

estrogen: One of a group of steroid hormones synthesized mainly in the ovaries responsible for female sexual development.

estrogen replacement therapy: A treatment using the synthetic form of estrogen to treat amenorrhea, symptoms of menopause, to aid in the prevention of osteoporosis and heart disease in women, and cancer of the prostate in men.

ethics: A system of morality, of right and wrong.

etiology: The study of the causes or origins of disease or injury.

euthanasia: The act of ending the life of a terminally ill patient who requests to die.

evaluation: The interpretation of a test.

evaporation: A method of heat transfer by which a liquid is converted into a gas.

eversion: The movement of the plantar aspect of the foot laterally, or away from the midline.

exacerbation: To increase the severity, to aggravate.

excision: The surgical removal of tissue.

exogenous: Arising from outside of the body.

exostosis: A bony outgrowth.

expectorant: A pharmacological agent used to "break up" phlegm by promoting coughing.

extension: A movement of a joint such that the angle formed by the two bones increases.

external rotation: To turn a body segment about its long axis so as to turn the anterior aspect of the segment toward the outside or laterally; also called lateral or outward rotation.

exteroreceptor: An afferent receptor in the skin or mucous membrane that responds to stimuli from outside the body.

extracorporeal lithotripsy: A noninvasive procedure to breakdown a kidney stone through the use of shock waves.

extradural anesthesia: *See* epidural anesthesia.

extrinsic: A term used to describe something originating from or outside an organ or body segment; opposite of intrinsic.

exudate: Accumulation of fluid with a high concentration of proteins, cells, or debris.

F

FABRE test (or FABER): Test for the hip involving Flexion, ABduction, External Rotation; also known as FABER or Patrick's test.

face validity: The extent to which a measure seems to test the outcome on your instincts (face value). The weakest measure of construct validity.

facial nerve: The seventh cranial nerve regulates facial movements, sensation, and taste on the anterior portion of the tongue. *See* Appendix 7.

facial palsy: Unilateral paralysis of the facial muscles caused by inflammation of a nerve.

factor analysis: A statistical procedure that analyzes the relationship of multiple variables and their contribution to the entire set of variables.

faint: Syncope, loss of consciousness due to insufficient blood flow to the brain.

false negative: A situation in which a patient is found not to have a disease or condition due to a faulty test procedure when in fact they do have the disease.

false positive: A situation in which a patient is found to have a disease or condition due to a faulty test procedure when in fact they do not have the disease.

familial: A term used to describe conditions that tend to "run in the family."

fartlek training: "Fartlek" from the Swedish word for "speed play"; a type of interval training that uses varied speeds and terrains.

fascia: A band of strong connective tissue that binds structures together.

fasciitis: Inflammation of the fascia covering the muscles.

fast twitch fiber: *See* type II fiber.

fat soluble vitamins: Vitamins A, D, E, and K.

fatigue: The inability to continue an exercise.

fatty acid: An important component of lipids; a long hydrocarbon chain with an even number of carbon atoms.

female athlete triad: A common combination of anorexia (or bulimia), amenorrhea, and osteoporosis.

femoral artery: The main artery that supplies blood to the legs, found most superficially in the femoral triangle.

femoral nerve: Nerve of the anterior thigh that innervates the quadriceps; it passes through the femoral triangle.

femoral nerve test: A traction test in which the patient is side-lying with affected side up and neck slightly flexed. The examiner extends the hip approximately 15 degrees with the knee extended followed by a flexing of the knee. Pain radiating into the anterior thigh is a positive test.

femoral triangle: A triangular shaped anatomical structure located in the anterior, proximal thigh bordered by the inguinal ligament and the sartorius and adductor longus muscles. The femoral nerve and artery pass through this triangle.

femur: The long bone of the thigh.

fibrillation: A rapid and irregular rhythm of the heart muscle fibers causing a lack of synchrony such that there is an inability to efficiently pump blood.

fibrin: The final product in the formation of a blood clot. The mesh-like substance is the product of fibrinogen.

fibrinogen: A substance found in the blood that when acted upon by thrombin produces fibrin.

fibroadenoma: A benign tumor of the breast.

fibrocartilage: A dense type of cartilage found between the vertebra and at the pubic symphysis.

fibrocystic breast disease: The most common cause of benign breast lumps.

fibroid: A benign uterine tumor.

fibroma: A benign tumor found in connective tissue.

fibrosis: Abnormal scar formation in connective tissue.

Finkelstein's test: A special test of the wrist to test for the presence of de Quervain's. *See* Special Tests—Hand/Wrist (Appendix 16).

first-class lever: A type of machine in which the axis is between the motive and resistive forces. Examples include pliers, scissors, and a teeter-totter. The advantage of a first-class lever depends on the relative length of the moment arms of the motive and resistive forces. In the human body there are few first-class levers. One example, however, is the action of the gastroc/soleus unit (motive force) at the ankle joint (axis) during a toe-standing motion (ground reaction force is the resistive).

first-order neuron: Afferent neurons in the periphery.

first ray: The first tarso metatarsal joint of the foot.

fissure: A groove or cleft-like defect.

fistula: An abnormal opening from an organ or structure.

fitness: A measure of one's strength, flexibility, and endurance.

fixation: A stabilization technique.

flaccidity: Decreased muscle tone.

flatulence: Abdominal or intestinal gas expelled through the anus.

flexibility: Mobility; the range of motion about a joint.

flexion (FLEX): The movement at a joint in which the segments of a joint are brought toward each other; a movement of a joint such that the angle formed by the two bones decreases.

flu: *See* Influenza.

fluidotherapy: A form of thermotherapy involving the use of very fine, dry particles flowing about the injured part.

fluoride: A mineral that helps prevent tooth decay.

fluoroscopy: An x-ray device that allows images to be seen directly on a fluorescent screen without the need for developing film.

folliculitis: Boils or blisters caused by the inflammation of hair follicles due to a bacterial infection.

foramen: An opening or hole in a bone.

force: A push or pull that causes or tends to cause a change in shape or motion and is measured in pounds or Newtons.

force arm: The perpendicular distance from the axis of rotation to the line of action of the force.

forward head: A posture characterized by positioning the head in an anterior position such that the neck exhibits a marked extension in the area of C4-C6. Often accompanies kyphosis and is a common cause of chronic neck and shoulder pain.

free nerve endings: Nociceptors; nerve endings that are particularly sensitive to mechanical, thermal, and chemical noxious stimuli.

frequency: The number of cycles, pulse repetitions per unit of time. Measured in hertz (Hz).

frequency distribution curve: The organization of test scores into intervals.

friction: The force resisting the "sliding" of one object past another.

frontal plane: Divides the body into dorsal and ventral or anterior and posterior parts. Motions that take place in this plane include abduction/adduction, radial/ulnar deviation, and lateral flexion of the trunk and head.

frostbite: Freezing or partial freezing of human tissue such as when exposed to prolonged or extreme cold.

functional assessment: Testing procedures that mimic the neuromuscular demands of various sports skills.

functional exercises: Exercises that require the patient to execute various activities that call upon the neuromuscular system to perform similarly to those activities involved in sport.

functional leg length: An assessment of leg length by comparing the height of the anterior superior iliac spine (ASIS) in the standing patient.

functional position: The act of placing a limb or joint in the position most appropriate or most used.

functional progression: A series of sport-specific and graduated exercises designed with the intent of returning the individual safely and efficiently to full participation.

furuncle: An inflammation of the skin containing pus caused by staphylococcus bacteria, which enters through a hair follicle or skin wound.

G

Gaenslen's: A special test of the sacroiliac joint. *See* Special Tests—Hip (Appendix 16).

gait: Walking pattern.

galactose: A form of sugar created from the breakdown of lactose.

gallbladder: A small organ (sac) just inferior to the liver, in which bile is stored.

gallstone: A hard mass made up of cholesterol, bile pigments, and/or calcium salts that is found in the gallbladder.

Galvanic electrical stimulation: Direct current electrical stimulation, named for Luigi Galvani (1737-1798), who was an Italian physician and physicist known for his electrical stimulation experiments of frog nerves and muscles.

Galveston Orientation and Amnesia Test (GOAT): A test that measures early recovery of memory and orientation to person, place, and time.

ganglion: A cyst-like structure that often forms in a tendon, commonly found in the wrist. An enlarged area in the posterior sensory root of a spinal nerve.

gangrene: Tissue death due to lack of blood supply.

gapping test: A special test of the sacroiliac joint. *See* Special Tests—Hip (Appendix 16).

gastrectomy: The surgical removal of the stomach or part of the stomach.

gastric acid: The digestive acid in the stomach that breaks down proteins.

gastric ulcer: A peptic ulcer.

gastrin: A hormone produced in the pyloric region of the stomach that stimulates the production of gastric acid.

gastritis: Inflammation of the lining of the mucous membrane of the stomach; causes may include virus, bacteria, alcohol, and drugs.

gastroenteritis: Inflammation of the stomach and intestines.

gate control theory: A theory of pain control based on the assumption that painful stimuli carried by Ad and C afferent nerves and sensory stimuli carried by Ab afferent nerves converge upon the dorsal horn in the substantia gelatinosa (SG). The larger Ab impulses travel faster and reach the SG and act to close the gate to the painful stimuli.

gene: The basic unit of DNA that controls the formation of a single polypeptide chain which determines the biochemical makeup of the proteins, rate of protein production, and the integration of protein into the cell structure.

gene therapy: An experimental medical procedure in which diseased or disease-causing genes are replaced by healthy ones.

generic drug: A drug name that indicates the class or type of compound.

genital herpes: Inflammation of the skin caused by the herpes simplex virus characterized by small blisters; transmitted through sexual contact.

genu: A sudden anatomical turn as in flexion; in orthopedics the term is used to denote the knee.

genu recurvatum: Hyperextending knees.

genu valgum: Literally means "knee turned outward," referring to the deformity in which the tibia is angled outward. The common term is "knock knees."

genu varum: Literally means "knee turned inward," referring to the deformity in which the tibia is angled inward. The common term is "bow-legged."

Gibney: Closed basket weave; a taping procedure for ankle mediolateral instability.

gingivectomy: Surgical removal of diseased tissue of the gums.

gingivitis: A build-up of plaque leading to inflammation of the gums.

gland: An organ responsible for secreting fluid either through specialized ducts (exocrine glands) or directly into the bloodstream (endocrine glands).

Glasgow coma scale: A means of assessing level of consciousness based on motor, verbal, and eye opening response.

Glasgow Coma Scale		
Eyes	spontaneously	4
	to verbal command	3
	to pain	2
	no response	1
Verbal	oriented and converses	5
	disoriented and converses	4
	inappropriate	3
	incomprehensible	2
	no response	1
Motor	obeys verbal command	6
	localizes painful stimulus	5
	normal flexion withdrawal	4
	decorticate posture	3
	decerebrate posture	2
	no response	1
	TOTAL	3-15

glaucoma: A disease of the eye in which increasing pressure in the eye can cause an eventual loss of sight if pressure is not controlled.

glenohumeral: The shoulder joint; the articulation between the head of the humerus and the glenoid fossa of the scapula.

gliding joint: A diarthrodial joint in which motion is created when the articular surfaces glide upon each other without axial motion.

glossopharyngeal nerve: Cranial nerve IX, responsible for swallowing and taste. *See* Appendix 7.

glucagon: A hormone produced by the pancreas that increases blood sugar by converting stored carbohydrates (glycogen) into glucose thus having the opposite effect of insulin.

glucose: A simple sugar, it is the main source of energy for the body and the sole source of energy for the brain; glucose is stored in the body as glycogen.

glucose tolerance test: A test for diabetes mellitus in which the concentration of sugar in the blood and urine are tested over a period of time in response to the intake of a known amount of glucose following a period of fasting.

glycogen: The stored form of glucose; stored in muscles and in the liver.

glycosuria: The presence of glucose in the urine.

Godfrey's sign: A special test for posterior cruciate ligament instability *See* Special Tests—Knee (Appendix 16).

goiter: Swelling in the throat, in particular the thyroid gland; causes include lack of iodine in the diet, or hyperthyroidism.

golfer's elbow: *See* medial epicondylitis.

golgi tendon organ (GTO): Mechanoreceptor that is sensitive to changes in length and tension. When the GTO is stimulated, it causes a reflex relaxation (autogenic inhibition) of the antagonist muscle(s).

gonadotropic hormones: One of the hormones released by the pituitary gland that stimulate activity in the ovaries and testicles.

goniometer: A protractor-like device used to measure joint angle.

gonorrhea: A common sexually transmitted disease caused by the bacterium *Neisseria gonorrhoeae* and characterized by painful urination and discharge from the penis or vagina.

gout: A disease that affects the joints, caused by excess uric acid in the joints; may also affect the kidneys.

graft: A procedure in which healthy tissue is used to replace diseased or damaged tissue.

grand mal: A convulsive type of seizure.

Graves' disease: An autoimmune disease that causes hyperthyroidism and a subsequent goiter and characteristic bulging eyes.

gravity: A motive force that is always present and acts on the center of gravity of every object. Acceleration caused by the force of gravity is 9.8 m/s^2 or 32 ft/s^2. In other words, an object that is dropped from a building will be traveling at a velocity of 9.8 m/s^2 exactly 1 second after it is released and 19.6 m/s^2 exactly 2 seconds after it is released, etc.

ground fault interrupters (GFI): An electrical safety device that will cause the electrical current to shut off if it detects leakage of current.

ground reaction force: The equal and opposite force applied by the ground in response to the force applied to the ground as in walking, running, jumping, etc.

Guillain-Barré syndrome: A disease affecting the peripheral nervous system causing inflammation, weakness, and loss of sensation in the arms and legs; appears 10 to 20 days after a respiratory infection.

gunstock deformity: A humeral condylar fracture.

H

half-value thickness: The depth of a tissue or substance at which the intensity of a beam of radiation will reach half of its original value.

halitosis: Bad breath.

hallucination: The perception of something that is not really there, for example, "seeing or hearing things."

hallux: Great toe.

hallux rigidus: A restriction of flexion/extension of the first metatarsophalangeal joint.

hallux valgus: Bunion; angling inward of the great toe.

Halstead's maneuver: A special test of the shoulder for thoracic outlet syndrome. *See* Special Tests—Shoulder (Appendix 16).

hammer toe: A flexion deformity of the toe, commonly the second toe.

hangman's fracture: A fracture of the pedicle of C2, sometimes accompanied by anterior dislocation of the body of C2.

hardening of the arteries: *See* arteriosclerosis.

harelip: *See* cleft lip.

Hawkins-Kennedy impingement test: A special test of the shoulder for impingement. *See* Special Tests—Shoulder (Appendix 16).

HDL: *See* high-density lipoprotein.

heart rate: The rate at which the heart "beats" in 1 minute.

heartburn: Caused by acid reflux, a recurrent burning sensation in the chest and throat.

heat cramps: Muscle spasm brought on by prolonged exposure to heat, humidity, and/or the presence of dehydration.

heat exhaustion: Heat illness brought on by prolonged exposure to heat, humidity, and/or the presence of dehydration. Symptoms include rapid pulse, pale skin, profuse sweating, and increased body temperature (rectal) to 102°F. Treatment includes immediate removal from heat and rapid oral and intravenous rehydration.

heat illness: One of the many forms of illness brought on by dehydration and/or exercising in excessive temperatures and humidity levels.

heat rash: Prickly heat; a local rash brought on by prolonged exposure to heat.

heat stroke: A serious, life-threatening form of heat illness brought on by prolonged exposure to heat, humidity, and/or the presence of dehydration. Symptoms include loss of consciousness; shallow breathing; rapid pulse; red, hot skin; mild to no sweating; and core temperature (rectal) of 106°F or higher. Treatment includes immediate removal from heat and rapid oral and intravenous rehydration.

heel counter: The portion of a shoe that encloses the calcaneus and provides rearfoot stabilization.

heel strike: The point at which the heel makes contact with the ground following the swing phase of the walking cycle.

Heimlich maneuver: A first aid technique used to dislodge a foreign object from a choking person's airway.

hemarthrosis: Bleeding and swelling in a joint.

hematemesis: Vomiting of blood.

hematocrit: The percentage of red blood cells in the total blood volume.

hematoma: The formation of a blood clot within the tissue, initially may appear as swelling.

hematuria: Blood in the urine.

hemiparesis: *See* hemiplegia.

hemiplegia: Paralysis affecting one side of the body. The face and upper extremity are often more affected.

hemodialysis: *See* dialysis.

hemoglobin: An iron-containing porphyrin responsible for the pigment in red blood cells and is responsible for carrying oxygen throughout the body.

hemolysis: The normal process in which red blood cells are broken down in the spleen.

hemophilia: An inherited disorder in which the blood clots too slowly leading to prolonged bleeding; caused by a lack of antihemophilic factor (factor VIII).

hemopoietic: Related to the formation of blood cells.

hemorrhage: Bleeding.

hemorrhoid: A distended vein at the opening of the anus caused by straining.

hemostasis: The normal clotting process which controls bleeding.

hemothorax: Blood in the pleural cavity between the chest wall and the lungs.

hepatic: Pertaining to the liver.

hepatitis: Inflammation of the liver; causes include alcohol abuse, drug use, viral infection, or poisons. Symptoms include fever, headache, nausea, and general weakness. Hepatitis A (infectious hepatitis) is transmitted through contaminated food or water; hepatitis B and C (serum hepatitis) are transmitted through sexual contact or contact with bodily fluids; hepatitis D is a form of hepatitis that only appears when hepatitis B virus is already present.

Herb's palsy: *See* Erb's palsy.

hereditary: Passing a genetic trait from parent to offspring.

hernia: Protrusion of an organ or tissue through an opening as in a weakening in the surrounding wall.

herniated vertebral disk: A condition in which the annulus fibrosis of the vertebral disc fails and the nucleus bulges or extrudes through the outer wall placing pressure on the spinal nerve roots. *See* disk injury.

herpes simplex: The simple form of the herpes virus, characterized by blisters on the face, mouth, or genitals.

herpes zoster: "Shingles," characterized by pain along the distribution of a nerve; *see also* chicken pox.

hertz (Hz): The SI unit of frequency.

hiccup: Involuntary spasm of the diaphragm along with the closing of the glottis, producing a "hiccup" sound.

high-density lipoprotein (HDL): Considered to be the "good cholesterol"; a specific protein in the blood thought to remove cholesterol, thereby protecting against heart disease.

high-voltage current: A type of electrical nerve stimulation that uses voltage greater than 150 volts with pulses of very short duration, commonly a twin peak pulse.

Hill-Sachs lesion: A defect in the posterior articular cartilage of the humeral head found after anterior dislocation of the shoulder.

HIPS: Systematic evaluation procedure consisting of History, Inspection, Palpation, and Special Tests. *See also* HOPS (observation instead of inspection).

histamine: A compound associated with mast cells that is released during allergic reactions, causes dilation of blood vessels and contraction of smooth muscle, especially the lungs causing a narrowing of the airway.

histamine blocker: A drug that inhibits the action of histamine; H1 blocker is used to treat inflammation; H2 blocker is used to block the production of stomach acid to treat peptic ulcers.

hirsutism: Excessive growth of hair in unusual places, especially in women.

HIV: *See* human immunodeficiency virus.

hives: The common term for an itchy rash resulting from an allergic reaction.

Hodgkin's disease: A malignant disease of the lymph nodes and spleen; symptoms include enlarged lymph nodes, fever, loss of appetite, and weight loss.

Hoffman's reflex (digital): Special tests for upper motor neuron lesion in which the examiner "flicks" the distal phalanx of the first, second, or third finger. A reflex flexion of the thumb or adjacent finger (not flicked) is a positive sign.

Homan's sign: A special test for deep vein thrombophlebitis. The patient's foot is passively dorsiflexed while the knee is extended.

homeostasis: The tendency of a system to maintain stability.

homogeneity of covariance: Equality of correlation among three or more repeated measures taken on the same subjects.

homogeneity of variance: Equality of variance among two or more measures.

Hoover's test: A special test used to test for malingering.

HOPS: Systematic evaluation procedure consisting of History, Observation, Palpation, and Special Tests. *See also* HIPS (inspection instead of observation).

hordeolum: *See* stye.

horizontal abduction: Movement away from the midline in the transverse plane.

horizontal adduction: Movement toward the midline in the transverse plane.

horizontal extension: An extension movement that takes place in the transverse (horizontal) plane.

horizontal flexion: A flexion movement that takes place in the transverse (horizontal) plane.

hormone: A substance produced by an endocrine gland and released into the blood stream which acts to control or modify an organ or tissue.

Hughston test: *See* jerk test of Hughston.

human immunodeficiency virus (HIV): The virus that causes AIDS; contracted through sexual intercourse or contact with infected blood.

human papilloma virus (HPV): A virus that causes various human warts to the hands, feet, genitals, and anus; some are associated with cancer.

hunting response: The vasodilation that follows the initial vasoconstriction after the application of cold.

hydrocele: Swelling of the scrotum.

hydrocephalus: "Water on the brain"; an abnormal increase in cerebrospinal fluid around the brain.

hydrocortisone: A corticosteroid used to treat inflammation and allergies.

hydrotherapy: The therapeutic use of water.

hyper: A prefix denoting an increase, excessive, above, or more than.

hyperabduction syndrome: Symptoms of thoracic outlet syndrome caused by abduction of the arm.

hyperemia: A collection of excess blood.

hyperextension: Extreme extension; beyond normal extension.

hyperglycemia: Abnormally high glucose levels caused by undiagnosed or improperly treated diabetes mellitus.

hyperhidrosis: Excessive sweating.

hypermobility: An abnormal increase in range of motion; excessive joint play; commonly referred to as "double-jointed." A sign of Marfan's and Ehlers-Danlos syndromes.

hyperopia: Far-sightedness.

hyperparathyroidism: Increased calcium levels in the blood and decreased calcium levels in bones caused by overactivity of the parathyroid glands.

hyperplasia: Hypertrophy; an increase in growth of cells.

hyperpnea: Hyperventilation.

hyperreflexia: An abnormal increase in normal reflex response.

hypertension: High blood pressure.

hyperthermia: Elevated body temperature; *see* heat illness.

hyperthyroidism: Overactivity of the thyroid gland.

hypertonic (hypertonus): An abnormal increase in muscle tone; a solution that has increased osmotic pressure.

hypertrophic cardiomyopathy: A thickening of the cardiac muscle walls causing arterial obstruction and leading to mitral valve prolapse and possible aortic rupture.

hypertrophy: Increase in the size of a tissue due to an enlargement of the cells rather than multiplication of cells.

hyperventilation: Rapid breathing characterized by a reduction in CO_2 in the blood.

hyphema: A collection of blood in the anterior chamber of the eye.

hypo: A prefix denoting a decrease or lack of; under; below.

hypoglossal nerve: Cranial nerve XII, responsible for swallowing and movements of the tongue. *See* Appendix 7.

hypoglycemia: A decrease in blood glucose; occurs in diabetes patients with an inadequate intake of carbohydrates.

hypoplasia: The failure of a tissue or organ to fully develop.

hyporeflexia: Decreased reflex.

hypotension: Abnormally low blood pressure.

hypothenar: The medial side of the "heel of the hand."

hypothermia: Body temperature below 95°F caused by prolonged exposure to cold temperatures.

hypothyroidism: Underactivity of the thyroid gland; symptoms include decreased heart rate, weight gain, and apathy.

hypotonic (hypertonus): An abnormal decrease in muscle tone; a solution that has decreased osmotic pressure.

hypoventilation: Abnormally slow breathing rate.

hypoxia: Decrease in oxygen supplied to the tissues.

hysterectomy: The surgical excision of the uterus.

iatrogenic: Referring to an illness or medical condition caused as a direct result of the treatment; a complication of a medical treatment.

idiopathic: Unknown cause.

Ila: Inferiolateral angle (of the sacrum).

ileostomy: A medical procedure whereby the ileum is brought through the abdominal wall to form a new opening (stoma).

ileum: The distal end of the small intestine leading to the large intestine.

iliotibial band (ITB) friction syndrome: A chronic injury caused by the friction created when the ITB rubs over the lateral femoral epicondyle. Common in running and cycling athletes. Also known as runner's knee; *see* Special Tests—Hip (Appendix 16).

ilium: One of the two large, flat, dish-shaped bones of the hip.

immune: A resistance to disease; not susceptible to a particular disease; possessing the antibodies to fight off a particular antigen.

immune system: The system including the thymus, spleen, and lymph nodes that protect the body from disease organisms and foreign substances.

immunology: The study of the immune system.

immunostimulant: A drug that increases the immune system and thus improves the body's ability to fight disease.

immunosuppressant: A drug that inhibits the immune system and thus prevents the body from attacking itself; commonly used to prevent rejection following organ transplant.

impedance (active electrode): The resistance in a tissue to the flow of electrical current.

impetigo: A bacterial skin infection that is highly contagious; caused by staphylococcal and sometimes streptococcal, occurs around the nose and mouth and rapidly spreads into patches of crusty pustules.

implant: A device or tissue surgically placed in the body.

impotence: A condition in which a male suffers from the inability to acquire or maintain an erection of the penis.

in situ: "In place"; refers to a disease that has remained localized.

in vitro: Literally means "in glass"; a test or procedure that is carried out in a laboratory setting, ie, not in a living being; the opposite of in vivo.

in vivo: Literally means "in the living body"; a test or procedure that occurs in a living being.

incision: A cut or wound caused by a sharp straight object such as in surgery.

incisor: One of the eight front teeth.

incontinence: Inability to control the release of urine or feces.

independent variable: A variable controlled by the research design that may have influence on other variables (ie, the dependent measure).

Index Medicus: An extensive medical index of the National Library of Medicine in which journal information is listed by subject, author, title, key words, journal, year, and country of publication.

indigestion: A feeling of discomfort following eating caused by abnormal digestion or ingestion of irritable foods.

inertia: The resistance to changes in movement.

infarction: The death of an organ due to loss of blood flow usually caused by a blood clot.

infection: Invasion of the body by a pathogen.

inferential: A type of research design in which inferences are made.

inflammation: The immediate response following injury that may be caused by mechanical, thermal, chemical, or infection; signs and symptoms include redness (rubor), pain (dolar), swelling (tumor), heat (calor), loss of function (functio laesa).

inflammatory bowel disease: Crohn's disease or ulcerative colitis.

inflammatory joint disease: Swelling, redness, and pain around a joint; any type of arthritis.

influenza: A highly contagious viral infection affecting the respiratory system. Symptoms include weakness, cough, fever, and muscle aches.

informed consent: A process by which a subject or patient is fully informed of the possible benefits and dangers of a medical procedure or participation in a research study and voluntarily agrees to participate.

infrared: The part of the electromagnetic spectra just before visible light; infrared modalities include ice, cold packs, cold whirlpool, vapocoolant sprays, warm whirlpool, hydroculator packs, and paraffin.

ingestion: To eat or drink; to take by mouth.

ingrown toenail: A painful condition in which the edge of the nail grows into the skin, commonly in one of the distal corners; caused by improper clipping of the toenail.

inguinal hernia: Protrusion of an organ or tissue through an opening at the inguinal canal.

inhaler: A pharmacologic agent in the form of a gas or vapor that is breathed into the lungs to treat conditions of the lungs, especially asthma.

inherited: A trait that is passed from parent to child.

injection: The act of using a syringe to inject a drug.

innominate bone: The hipbone consisting of the ilium, ishium, and pubis.

insemination: Injection of semen into the vagina.

insertion: The muscle attachment nearest the trunk.

insomnia: Inability or difficulty sleeping.

instability: In orthopedic assessment, the state of a joint when the ligaments fail to support it.

insulin: A protein hormone produced in the pancreas important in regulating the absorption of glucose and thus controlling blood sugar levels; diabetes is the inability to produce the hormone or adequate amounts of the hormone and is treated with insulin injections.

intensity: (In modalities) amplitude; the rate at which energy is delivered.

interclass correlation (interclass reliability coefficient): An estimation of reliability that uses correlational procedures.

interferential: A type of electrical stimulation in which two channels of differing frequencies "interfere" with each other, causing periods of constructive and destructive interference, creating a "beat" frequency equal to the difference between the two frequencies (ie, channel A at a frequency of 4000 and channel B at a frequency of 4010 produce a beat frequency of 10 Hz).

internal fixation: A method of stabilizing a fracture with surgically placed screws, rods, and plates.

internal rotation: A rotation movement so as to turn the anterior aspect of the segment toward the inside or medially; medial rotation; inward rotation.

interneuron: A neuron in the central nervous system that acts as a link between two neurons.

interoreceptor: An afferent receptor in the skin or mucous membrane that responds to stimuli from within the body such as tissue tension or chemical changes.

interosseous membrane: The connective tissue between two or more bones.

interstitial: A space between tissues or body parts.

interstitial cystitis: Inflammation of the lining of the bladder.

intertrigo: Skin chafing.

intervertebral disks: A broad, flexible, fibrocartilagenous disk found between each vertebrae that functions to

connect the vertebrae, provide cushioning, and promote movement between vertebrae; made up of a
fibrous outer layer called the annulus fibrosis and a gel-
like inner layer called the nucleus pulposis; *see also* herniated disk.

intestine: The continuation of the alimentary canal, from
the stomach to the anus, divided first into the small
intestine (duodenum, jejunum, ileum) and then the
large intestine (cecum, vermiform appendix, colon, rectum).

**intraclass correlation (ICC; intraclass reliability coeffi-
cient):** An estimation of reliability that uses analysis of
variance.

intractable: A disease that does not respond to treatment.

intramedullary rod: A long metal rod that is placed into
the medulla of a fractured bone.

intraocular pressure: The pressure created by fluid levels
in the eye.

intravenous: Pertaining to the inside of a vein.

intrinsic: A term used to describe something originating
from and located within an organ or body segment;
opposite of extrinsic.

invasive: A medical procedure in which an instrument is
introduced into the body tissues through the skin or
body orifice; a tumor or microorganism that spreads
throughout body tissues.

inversion: Of the foot, motion of the foot so as to turn the
sole of the foot inward.

inversion stress test: The inversion force of the talar tilt
test, a test in which the ankle is inverted to assess the
lateral ligaments of the ankle.

involuntary: A situation in which the individual did not
provide informed consent.

inward rotation: A rotation movement so as to turn the
anterior aspect of the segment toward the inside or
medially; medial rotation; internal rotation.

iodine: A nonmetallic element with several uses including as a contrast or stain for testing, as a topical antiseptic, and as a treatment for thyroid disease.

ion: Electrically charged atom.

iontophoresis: The use of electrical stimulation (direct current) to drive ions to deeper tissues.

ipsilateral: Denoting the same side.

iris: The colored part of the eye, responsible for the regulation of light that enters the eye by the muscular ring formed around the pupil.

iron: A metallic element that occurs in the important biological substances such as the heme of hemoglobin, myoglobin, and certain other enzymes; iron deficiency leads to anemia; meat and liver are good dietary sources of iron; the recommended daily intake is 10 g (males)/12 g (females).

irrigation: The cleansing of a wound by flushing it with water, saline antiseptic or other solution.

irritable bowel syndrome: Abnormal muscle contractions of the bowel causing abdominal pain and irregular bowel movements (diarrhea or constipation). There appears to be no physiological cause and there is no deterioration of general health. Often occurs due to stress or anxiety.

ischemia: Reduced oxygen supply to a tissue commonly due to constriction of blood vessels or edema.

isokinetic: A type of resistance exercise characterized by accommodating resistance throughout the full range of motion at a preset velocity (ie, the velocity remains constant while resistance varies according to the force output of the individual).

isometric: Literally means "same length" and refers to the length of the muscle. Isometric resistance exercise is characterized by a development of tension in a muscle without movement of related joints. Often used during periods of immobility to reduce atrophy.

isotonic: Literally means "same tension," however, in biomechanics it refers to resistance exercise in which concentric and eccentric exercises are performed against a constant weight.

itis: Suffix meaning "inflammation of."

Jackson's compression test: Special test of the cervical spine for nerve root compression. *See* Special Tests—Spine (Appendix 16).

JAT: Abbreviation for *Journal of Athletic Training*, the official journal of the National Athletic Trainer's Association.

jaundice: A condition characterized by a yellowing of the skin and whites of the eyes; excessive excretion of bilirubin by the liver, a common sign of liver disease.

jerk test of Hughston: A special test of the knee for the presence of ACL injury similar to the pivot shift test. The examiner applies a medial rotation force to the lower leg with the knee flexed to 90 degrees. Between 20 to 30 degrees the tibia shifts anteriorly and is reduced at full extension.

Jobe relocation test: A special test for shoulder instability. *See* Special Tests—Shoulder (Appendix 16).

jock itch: *See* tinea cruris.

joint capsule: The fibrous tissue surrounding and providing stability to a joint.

joint mobilization: A manual therapy used to improve the accessory motions of sliding, spinning, and rolling.

joint play: The accessory movement that is necessary for physiological motion to occur; the amount of sliding, spinning, and rolling motion available in a joint.

joint position sense: The ability to detect actively or passively placed joint positions; a measure of proprioception.

Jones fracture: A transverse stress fracture of the fifth metatarsal.

JOSPT: Abbreviation for *Journal of Orthopedic and Sports Physical Therapy.*

joule: The international unit of work, energy; equal to the amount of work needed to move 1 Newton a distance of 1 meter or the work needed for 1 ampere to flow through the resistance of 1 ohm.

JRC-AT (Joint Review Committee for Athletic Training): The professional review committee of the Commission on Accreditation of Allied Health Education Programs for athletic training.

JSR: Abbreviation for *Journal of Sport Rehabilitation*.

jumper's knee: The common term for tendinitis of the patella tendon.

Karnofsky scale: A rating used to determine a person's usual activities; used to evaluate progress.

Kehr's sign: Referred pain to the left shoulder from diaphragm or spleen injury or disease.

keloid: A firm, nodular scar formation with irregular bands of collagen that forms as a result of abnormal healing following an incision or burn.

Kendall test: A special test for rectus femoris tightness. *See* Special Tests—Hip (Appendix 16).

keratin: A scleroprotein found in nails and hair.

keratitis: Inflammation of the cornea.

keratosis: One of a number of abnormal, warty, pigmented growths on the skin, generally benign, however actinic keratosis may develop into squamous cell carcinoma if untreated.

Kernig sign: Special test of the spine for nerve root compression or irritation of the dura mater. *See* Special Tests—Spine (Appendix 16).

ketoacidosis (ketosis): Enhanced production of ketones sometimes occurring as a complication of diabetes mellitus.

kicker's knee: *See* patella tendonitis; also known as jumper's knee.

kidney stone: A hard, pebble-like mass commonly composed of calcium oxylate; also referred to as calculus; can be present in the kidney, ureter, or bladder causing severe pain (renal colic); in some cases must be removed surgically.

kilo: The SI unit for 1000.

kilocalorie (Kcal): A unit of measure for energy; equal to a nutritional calorie.

kinanesthesia: Inability to sense joint motions or positions.

kinematics: The study of the time and space factors related to motion.

kinesiology: The study of human movement.

kinesthesia: A sense of motion, velocity and acceleration; kinesthesia is measured by "threshold to detection of passive movement."

kinesthetic awareness: The "sense" of body position or awareness, without which we would be unable to function with eyes closed.

kinetics: The study of the forces that cause motion.

Kleiger's test: A special test of the ankle ligaments. *See* Special Tests—Foot/Ankle (Appendix 16).

Klumpke palsy: A birth defect in which there is a lesion to the lower trunk of the brachial plexus or the nerve roots from C8-T1, causing weakness or paralysis of all ulnar innervated muscles as well as some of the distal median and radial innervated muscles.

kyphosis: The posterior curvature of the thoracic spine; increased kyphosis is often associated with a forward head posture and the cause of chronic neck and shoulder pain.

labyrinthitis: Inflammation of the labyrinth (inner ear) responsible for balance; can cause vertigo.

laceration: A torn or ragged open wound caused by blunt trauma.

Lachman's test: A special test of the knee for anterior cruciate injury. *See* Special Tests—Knee (Appendix 16).

lacrimation: An excess secretion of tears.

lactic acid: A byproduct of glucose metabolism in the absence of sufficient oxygen.

lactose: The disaccharide found in dairy milk.

lactose intolerance: A condition marked by the inability to break down and absorb the sugar lactose causing cramping and diarrhea.

lamina: The posterior arch of vertebrae that connects the spinous process to the pedicle.

laminectomy: The surgical removal of the lamina of the spine, usually to gain access to a ruptured disc.

laparoscope: An instrument used to examine the abdominal cavity.

large intestine: The distal end of the alimentary canal between the small intestine and the anus consisting of the cecum, vermiform appendix, and colon.

Larsen-Johansson disease: Similar to Osgood-Schlatter disease, it is an apophysitis at the inferior pole of the patella.

laryngectomy: The surgical removal of all or part of the larynx, usually as a treatment for cancer.

laryngitis: Inflammation of the larynx causing one to "lose his or her voice."

larynx: The organ between the pharynx and trachea that produces sound and prevents food from entering the airway.

Lasegues test: Special test of the Lumbar spine for nerve root compression. *See* Special Tests—Spine (Appendix 16).

laser (light amplification by stimulated emission of radiation): A form of treatment for surgery, cauterization, and treatment of skin wounds.

lateral: Toward the side.

lateral epicondylitis: Often caused by the repeated deceleration force of slowing the racket after hitting a tennis ball.

lateral flexion: A flexion movement of the trunk or neck toward one side.

lateral rotation: A rotation movement so as to turn the anterior aspect of the segment toward the outside or laterally; external rotation; outward rotation.

lateral spinothalmic tract: The tract or path of the spinal cord where Ad and C neurons synapse and send noxious stimuli to the brain.

Law of Grothus and Draper: Energy that is not absorbed will be transmitted to deeper tissues.

laxative: A pharmacological agent used to treat constipation or to clear the intestines prior to diagnostic procedures.

laxity: The state of being loose; the amount of joint play or joint movement.

LDL: *See* low-density lipoprotein.

left rotation: A rotation of the trunk or neck toward the left.

leg length discrepancy: A measurable difference in bilateral leg length. Commonly measured as true leg length or real leg length; *see also* functional leg length and apparent leg length.

Legg-Calvé-Perthes disease: Coxa plana, or osteochondritis deformans juvenilis; a vascular necrosis of the proximal femoral epiphysis occurring in boys 3 to 12 years of age.

Legionnaire's disease: A respiratory infection often leading to pneumonia that can be contracted through air-conditioning or water; named after the nationally publicized breakout at an American Legion convention in 1976.

lesion: Any wound or injury; pathologic changes in a tissue.

leukemia: A proliferation of abnormal leukocytes affecting the production of normal white blood cells, red blood cells, and platelets; there are several varieties of leukemia.

leukocytes: White blood cells.

leukoplakia: Potentially cancerous white patches that develop in the mouth, vagina, or on the penis.

lever arm: *See* force arm.

lichen planus: Flat-topped, shiny eruptions found on male genitalia, flexor surfaces of the skin, and in the mouth that resolve spontaneously, sometimes months or years after their first appearance.

ligament: A tough, fibrous connective tissue that joins two or more bones at a joint.

Likert scale: A scale used to measure an individual's level of agreement or disagreement with a statement using a 3- or 5-point scale. Example: strongly disagree, disagree, neutral, agree, strongly agree.

linea alba: The median longitudinal tendinous line along the abdomen from the xiphoid to the pubic symphysis separating the two rectus abdominis muscles.

lipidosis: An abnormality of lipid metabolism that is hereditary in which fats are not properly broken down and thus there is an accumulation of lipids.

lipids: A group of fats that are stored in the body and used later for energy; they are important due to their association with vitamins and essential fatty acids.

lipoma: A benign fatty tumor.

lipoproteins: Important for the transport of lipids; one of many proteins that combine with lipids found in blood plasma and lymph.

liposarcoma: A malignant tumor of fatty tissue.

liposuction: A surgical procedure in which fat is removed by suction.

lipotropin: A substance in the anterior pituitary gland that stimulates the transport of stored fat to the bloodstream.

Lisfranc joint: The tarsometatarsal joints; articulation of the five metatarsal bases with the tarsal bones.

Lisfranc's fracture: A fracture and or displacement of one or more tarsometatarsal joints.

Lisinopril: An ACE inhibitor used to treat hypertension, heart failure, and acute myocardial infarction. Examples include Zestril (Zeneca Pharmaceuticals, Lincoln University, Pa) and Prinivil (Merck & Co, Inc, Whitehouse Station, NJ).

little league elbow: *See* medial epicondylitis.

liver: Large gland found in the upper right quadrant responsible for many vital functions such as synthesizing bile; metabolizing carbohydrates, proteins, and fats; controlling blood sugar by converting glucose to glycogen; and removing excess amino acids.

load-shift test: A special test of the shoulder in which the humeral head is gently pushed into the glenoid fossa and anterior and posterior translation is applied.

LOC: Abbreviation for " loss of consciousness."

local anesthesia: A method of preventing pain by injecting a drug into or around a nerve, thereby reducing the loss of sensation in the area supplied by that nerve.

locomotor system: All of the components of the body segments responsible for moving the body as a whole.

long thoracic nerve: The nerve supplying the serratus anterior, it arises from C5-7; injury to the long thoracic nerve results in characteristic "winging scapula" due to the inability to stabilize the scapula with the serratus anterior.

longitudinal arch: The medial arch of the foot; *see* arch.

longitudinal axis: An imaginary line along the length of a body.

loose (open) packed position: A joint position when the bone ends in a position of least congruency. In this position, the joint will exhibit the most laxity.

lordosis: The anterior curve of the lumbar spine.

Lou Gehrig's disease: *See* amyotrophic lateral sclerosis.

low dye technique: A taping procedure for the longitudinal arch.

low-density lipoprotein (LDL): The "bad" cholesterol; a lipoprotein that carries cholesterol in the blood; high levels of LDL are associated with heart disease and atherosclerosis.

lower motor neuron lesion (LMNL): A spinal cord lesion resulting in hyporeflexia, decrease in tone, or complete paralysis. Neuropraxia, axonotmesis, and neurotmesis are examples of LMNLs.

low-voltage current: Electrical stimulation using currents less than 150 volts.

Ludington's test: A special test of the shoulder to assess the integrity of the biceps tendon. A positive test indicates complete rupture of the biceps tendon. *See* Special Tests—Shoulder (Appendix 16).

lumbago: A term describing lower back pain.

lumbar spine: The last five vertebrae proximal to the sacrum.

lupus: *See* systemic lupus erythematosus.

lupus erythematosus: An autoimmune disease characterized by chronic inflammation of connective tissue; can cause arthritis and progressive kidney damage.

luxation: Dislocation.

Lyme disease: A debilitating disease caused by the bacteria transmitted from a tick; signs and symptoms initially include flu-like symptoms followed by a characteristic "bulls-eye" lesion and rash, general malaise, and fatigue. If progression is not stopped, neurological changes including peripheral neuropathy, insomnia, and memory loss will occur. The end stages are characterized by symptoms similar to rheumatoid arthritis. Named for the location where it was first discovered, Lyme, Conn.

lymph: The clear, yellowish fluid in the lymphatic system that contains lymphocytes, otherwise similar to plasma with fewer proteins; contains white blood cells and antibodies that help fight against the spread of infection playing an important role in the immune system.

lymphadenopathy: Swollen lymph nodes.

lymphatic system: The system made up of lymphatic vessels responsible for draining lymphatic fluid back into the blood.

lymph node: One of many small oval glands located along the lymphatic vessels.

lymphoma: A malignant tumor found in lymphoid tissue.

maculae: A spot; a small colored area.

magnetic resonance imaging (MRI): A technique that uses magnetic fields and radio frequencies to produce precise, high quality, cross-sectional images of the body.

main effects: In research, when a difference greater than that which could be expected due to error occurs across all levels of one of the factors.

malacia: Abnormal softening of a tissue.

malaise: Illness, discomfort.

malignant: A condition that is resistant to treatment and is characterized by uncontrolled growth, such as with cancer.

malingering: The act of pretending to be ill or injured, in order to be released from work or to gain attention.

mallet finger: A rupture of the extensor tendon causing a flexion of the DIP.

mammography: Imaging techniques including radiographic, ultrasound, and MRI techniques used for the diagnosis of breast disease.

mammoplasty: Any type of breast surgery or reconstruction including reduction, enlargement, and reconstruction after a mastectomy.

mandible: The bone of the lower jaw.

manic-depressive disorder: Bipolar disorder; a mental disorder in which the individual suffers from a shift between the two extremes of very high emotional "highs" and very low emotional "lows."

manipulation: A small amplitude, high force, passive therapy at the end range of motion for the purpose of restoring motion or improving position.

Mann-Whitney U: A nonparametric test of significance.

manual muscle testing (MMT): A form of resistive range of motion in which the examiner attempts to isolate individual muscles. *See* Muscle Grading (Appendix 13).

manual therapy: Therapeutic modalities that involve a "hands-on" approach. Joint mobilization and muscle energy are examples of manual therapy techniques.

march fracture: A stress fracture of a metatarsal; was commonly found in soldiers caused by prolonged marching.

Marfan's syndrome: A rare genetic connective tissue disorder that affects connective tissue; characterized by abnormally long bones, concave chest, pes planus, and generalized joint hypermobility. A severe complication of aortic dilation and weakness may cause aneurysm to develop. Mitral valve prolapse is associated with this syndrome. Patient should be referred to physician and monitored very closely.

mass: The amount of matter; a measure of inertia.

mast cell: A large connective tissue cell containing heparin, histamine, and serotonin, important in the inflammatory process.

mastectomy: A surgical removal of all or part of the breast; *see also* modified radical mastectomy and radical mastectomy.

mastitis: Inflammation of the breast.

maxilla: A bilateral bone that forms half of the upper jaw and face as well as the roof of the mouth.

maximal voluntary contraction (MVC): The maximal amount of force possible exerted against a static force.

Maximum compression test: Special test of the cervical spine for nerve root compression. *See* Special Tests—Spine (Appendix 16).

McConnell taping: Taping procedures designed to realign body structures; the most common procedure is used to treat patellofemoral dysfunction.

McKenzie extension exercises: Back and trunk exercises that emphasize extension with the intent of relieving pressure on the posterior wall of the disk.

McMurray's test: A special test of the knee to assess the presence of a meniscal tear. *See* Special Tests—Knee (Appendix 16).

mean: A statistical measure, the arithmetic average.

measles: A viral illness affecting primarily children, causing a characteristic rash and a fever; most Americans are inoculated against measles, mumps, and rubella (German measles).

mechanical advantage (MA): A situation in which a muscle is placed in a position such that it has an advantage due to the biomechanical arrangement. Such factors which affect mechanical advantage include muscle length, length of lever arm, and length of moment arm relative to the moment arm of the resistive force.

mechanical efficiency: The positioning of a limb or the body in such a way as to use the least energy in performing a given motion or to place the organ/tissue in a position of maximum advantage.

mechanoreceptor: A neuroreceptor that responds to mechanical stimuli such as touch, pressure, and tension.

medial: Toward the middle.

medial epicondylitis: Often caused by the repeated forceful contractions during a flexion motion and/or flexion/pronation motion such as that during a pitch (little league elbow).

medial rotation: A rotation movement so as to turn the anterior aspect of the segment toward the inside or medially; internal rotation; inward rotation.

medial tibial stress syndrome: Also known as shin splints; an overuse syndrome of the muscles in the deep posterior compartment of the leg; often associated with pes planus and pronated feet.

median (Mdn): The middle score, the 50th percentile.

median nerve: One of the terminal branches of the brachial plexus arising from the nerve roots C5-T1. The median nerve crosses the wrist through the carpal tunnel and is affected by compression in carpal tunnel syndrome.

mediolateral: From medial to lateral.

MEDLINE: The online version of *Index Medicus,* it is a bibliographic database covering the fields of medicine, nursing, dentistry, veterinary medicine, the health care system, and the preclinical sciences containing over 4070 biomedical journals and over 11 million citations from 1960 to the present.

medulla: The bone marrow containing center of a longitudinal bone; the inner part of an organ, particularly the kidneys, adrenal gland, and lymph nodes; the distal end of the brainstem referring to the medulla oblongata.

melanin: The dark pigmentation of the skin, hair, and eyes.

melanoma: Malignant neoplasm that can form melanin most commonly in skin, but frequently metastasizes to the lungs, lymph nodes, liver, and brain.

menarche: The onset of menstruation.

Meniere's disease: An inner ear disorder causing hearing loss, tinnitus, and dizziness.

meninges: The membranes of the spinal cord and brain (arachnoid, dura, and pia matters).

meningitis: Inflammation of the meninges; caused by bacterial or viral infection (bacterial is life-threatening while viral is often milder).

meniscectomy: The surgical removal or partial removal of the meniscus (usually of the knee).

meniscus: A crescent-shaped fibrocartilagenous in joints that helps to reduce friction; found in the knee, and temporomandibular, sternoclavicular, and acromioclavicular joints.

menopause: The termination of menses.

menstruation: The cyclical (approximately monthly) occurrence in women that involves the endometrial shedding (the lining of the uterus).

mesomorph: A somatotype (ie, body type) commonly termed the "athletic build."

metabolic rate: How quickly the body uses energy.

metabolism: The chemical and physical processes that occur in the body and enable it to function and grow.

metabolite: Any product of metabolism.

metacarpals: The long bones of the hand just distal to the carpals and proximal to the phalanges.

metaphysis: The growing portion of a long bone found between the diaphysis and the epiphysis.

metastasis: The infiltration or spreading of cancer to another part of the body; as a noun it refers to a tumor that has occurred through this process.

metatarsals: The long bones of the foot just distal to the tarsals and proximal to the phalanges.

microbe: *See* microorganism.

microbiology: The study of microorganisms.

microcurrent electrical nerve stimulator (MENS): A type of electrical stimulator that delivers electrical current less than 1000 mA. Efficacy of MENS is inconclusive.

microorganism: Any microscopic, single-celled organism.

microsurgery: Surgery performed with the use of a microscope.

mid stance: The mid point of the weightbearing phase of the walking cycle between heel strike and toe off.

migraine: A severe, often unilateral headache, usually accompanied by photophobia, phonophobia, nausea, vomiting, and dizziness.

mild brain injury (MBI): Concussion; brief loss of consciousness or a dazed feeling which can lead to post-concussion syndrome.

milliamp: Milliampere, one-thousandth of 1 ampere; unit of measure for electrical current.

mineral: An inorganic substance that serves as an important part of a healthy diet including potassium, calcium, sodium, phosphorus, and magnesium.

miotic: Drug-induced pupil constriction.

mitosis: The reproductive process of cell division.

mitral stenosis: A narrowing of the mitral valve causing the left atrium to work harder; an audible snap during diastole followed by a murmur can be heard during auscultation.

mitral valve: The valve in the heart that allows blood to flow from the left atrium to ventricle and prevents backflow.

mitral valve prolapse: A deformation of the mitral valve in the heart causing "a leak"; an audible murmur, chest pain, and abnormal heart rhythm are common.

MMR: Vaccination against measles, mumps, and rubella.

mobilization: The process of making a joint move more freely.

modality: A therapeutic agent used to reduce pain, swelling, and muscle spasm for the distinct purpose of promoting function.

mode: An approach to a treatment; in statistics, the score in a distribution that occurs most frequently.

modified radical mastectomy: A treatment for breast cancer similar to a radical mastectomy except the modified mastectomy leaves the pectoral muscles intact.

modified Romberg: A modification of the original Romberg test in which the patient is asked to stand on the limb of interest and maintain balance for a period of time (usually 20 to 30 seconds). This test is often performed with eyes closed in the case of assessing neuromuscular control following lower extremity injury.

modulation: In therapeutic modalities; the intentional alteration of one or more parameters in order to reduce the effect of accommodation

mole: Nevus; a brown spot on the skin.

molecule: The smallest quantity of a substance that still retains its chemical properties.

moment arm: *See* force arm.

mononucleosis: An acute infection caused by the Epstein-Barr virus in which there are large numbers of mononuclear leukocytes; symptoms include lethargy, fever, sore throat, and inflamed lymph nodes; the spleen can become enlarged with mononucleosis and persist up to 6 months.

monophasic current: An electrical current that does not cross the isoelectric line (ie, does not change polarity); has only one phase.

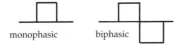

monophasic   biphasic

morbidity: Characteristic of illness or disease; the ratio of sick to healthy individuals in a given area.

morning sickness: A common occurrence of nausea and vomiting experienced early in a pregnancy.

mortality: A fatality; the state of being mortal; the death rate within a given population.

Morton's neuroma: A benign tumor on the common plantar nerve between the second and third or third and fourth metatarsal heads.

motive force: A force that causes motion. When lifting a weight against gravity, the muscles provide the motive force while gravity provides a resistive force. When lowering a weight with gravity, gravity provides the motive force, while the muscles provide a resistive force.

motor control: The neurophysiological factors that affect human movement, specifically the interaction between the brain and musculoskeletal system during performance of isolated tasks.

motor development: The study of changes in motor behavior over the entire life span.

motor learning: The study of the processes involved in learning and mastering new skills.

motor development: An efferent nerve cell that sends signals from the central nervous system to a muscle.

motor unit: An alpha motor neuron, its axon, and all the muscle fibers attached to it.

MS: *See* multiple sclerosis.

mucous membrane: Mucosa, the moist lining of many tubular structures consisting of an epithelial layer that contains secreting glands and deeper layers of connective tissue.

mucus: A clear secretion produced by mucous membranes that forms a protective barrier that lubricates and carries enzymes.

multiarticulate: Referring to the crossing of multiple joints. For example, the biceps brachii is considered multiarticulate due to the fact that it crosses and performs a function at the shoulder joint (shoulder flexion), radioulnar joint (supination), and ulnohumeral joint (elbow flexion).

multiple regression: A regression analysis on one dependent variable and multiple independent variables.

multiple sclerosis (MS): A demyelinating disease that affects the central nervous system. Patients suffer cycles of relapse followed by remission.

mumps: A common viral infection primarily affecting children that causes fever, nausea, vomiting, and characteristic inflammation of salivary glands; immunity is usually developed through a childhood infection.

murmur: A characteristic abnormal blood flow sound heard during auscultation.

Murphy's sign: A special test for lunate injury. *See* Special Tests—Hand/Wrist (Appendix 16).

muscle energy techniques: A treatment technique used to improve function by directing the concentrated muscular efforts of the patient at precise positions.

muscle relaxants: A pharmacologic agent used to reduce tension in the muscles.

muscle spindles: A stretch-sensitive receptor.

muscle strength: The maximum tension that can be produced by a muscle or muscle group.

muscle testing: *See* manual muscle testing.

muscle tone: A normal state of tension in a muscle that is controlled by reflex activity.

muscle wasting: Atrophy, the degeneration of a muscle.

muscular dystrophy (MD): An inherited disease in which there is marked muscle wasting. There are several variations of the disease; Duchenne's dystrophy is the most common; affecting primarily young boys.

muscular endurance: The ability of a muscle to contract repeatedly.

musculocutaneous nerve: One of the terminal branches of the brachial plexus arising from the nerve roots C5-C7. The musculocutaneous nerve innervates the biceps brachii and the coracobrachialis muscles.

MVC: *See* maximal voluntary contraction.

myalgia: Muscular pain.

myasthenia gravis: A disease in which there is marked weakness and fatigability of the muscles. Drooping of the upper eyelid is a common sign. Adolescent and young adult females are most often affected.

mycosis: A fungal disease.

myelin sheath: The outer covering, made of fat and protein, that surrounds and protects some nerves and improves conduction velocity.

myelitis: Inflammatory disease of the spinal cord common in multiple sclerosis but can occur in its absence; symptoms include headache, fever, muscle stiffness, pain, weakness, and eventually complete paralysis below the level of the disease; also refers to inflammation of the bone marrow (osteomyelitis).

myelocele: A neural tube defect; a severe form of spina bifida in which there is a protrusion of the meninges surrounding the spinal cord and the spinal cord and nerves roots are exposed.

myeloma: A tumor consisting of blood cells from bone marrow.

myelomalacia: A softening of the spinal cord.

myelosclerosis: Myelofibrosis; sclerosis of the bone marrow affecting the production of blood and its components.

myocardial infarction (MI): Commonly called a heart attack; a sudden insufficiency of blood and oxygen to an area of the heart causing tissue necrosis.

myocarditis: Inflammation of the heart muscle; can be caused by drugs, a virus, or radiation.

myocardium: Heart muscle.

myofascial release (MFR): A manual therapy in which deep friction massage is used to improve the mobility of fascial and muscular tissues.

myopathy: A muscle disease, usually one that results in muscle atrophy.

myopia: A condition commonly known as near-sightedness; it is caused by visual images coming into focus in front of the retina, resulting in blurred vision especially of objects at a distance.

myositis: Inflammation of a muscle or muscles causing pain and loss of strength.

myositis ossificans: Inflammation of a muscle leading to ossification within the muscle. A common complication to severe thigh contusions.

N

Naproxen: Naprosyn; a nonsteroidal anti-inflammatory medication.

narcolepsy: A disorder that causes uncontrollable episodes of falling asleep during the day.

narcosis: A drug-induced stupor or sleepiness.

narcotic: A substance with addictive properties known for its ability to dull the senses. A narcotic analgesic, for example, blocks the transmission of pain.

nares: Openings in the nose.

nasal septum: The cartilage/bone central divider of the nasal passage.

nasopharynx: The passageway from the nasal passage to the back of the throat.

nates: The buttocks.

natural immunity: Immunity to a disease by virtue of belonging to a particular race or species or an acquired immunity due to exposure to infection.

nausea: A sick feeling characterized by the need to vomit.

necrosis: Tissue death.

Neer's impingement test: A special test of the shoulder used to assess the presence of impingement. *See* Special Tests—Shoulder (Appendix 16).

neoplasm: An abnormal growth; tumor.

nephrectomy: The surgical removal of a kidney.

nephritis: Inflammation of the kidney.

nephroblastoma: "Wilm's tumor"; a fast-growing tumor of the kidneys affecting primarily children under 4 years old and rarely seen in children over the age of 18.

nephrolithotomy: Surgical removal of a kidney stone.

nephrology: The study of kidney disease.

nephron: The active filtering unit of the kidneys.

nephrosclerosis: A "hardening of the arteries" of the kidneys associated with hypertension.

nephrostomy: The surgical placement of a catheter directly to the kidney through the skin.

nerve: A bundle of fibers that transmit electrical impulses to and from the brain body tissues. Afferent nerves convey sensory information from the periphery to the brain while efferent nerves convey impulses from the brain to the periphery, especially muscles to provide motor function.

nerve block: A procedure used to reduce pain by injecting a local anesthetic into or around a nerve causing local analgesia.

nerve cell: A neuron; a specialized cell (composed of a cell body or soma, an axon, and one or more dendrites) that transmits electrical impulses from one area of the body to another.

nerve compression: Injury to a nerve induced by pressure, causing pain, weakness, or paresthesia.

neuralgia: A severe, sharp, or deep pain that follows a nerve distribution.

neurapraxia: Commonly referred to as a burner, stinger, or pinched nerve; a transient nerve compression or stretch causing pain, paresthesia, and weakness.

neuritis: Inflammation of a nerve, characterized by pain, numbness, or paresthesia.

neurogenic: Caused by or related to nerve injury.

neurogenic pain: Pain caused by injury to or illness of the nervous system.

neuroma: A benign tumorous growth from the fibrous covering of a peripheral nerve.

neuromuscular: Pertaining to the interaction and coordination of the nervous and muscular systems.

neuromuscular control: The efferent responses to the sensory information provided by kinesthesia and proprioception.

neuromuscular electrical stimulator (NMES): A type of electrical modality designed specifically to produce muscular contraction used to re-educate, strengthen, or maintain strength during periods of immobility, and to reduce spasticity.

neuron: Another term for a nerve cell; a specialized cell of the nervous system that carries information to and from the central nervous system, composed of a cell body (soma), an axon, and one or more dendrites.

neuropathy: Disease or injury to peripheral nerves causing pain, numbness, and weakness.

neuropraxia: A lower motor neuron lesion.

neurosis: A psychological disorder in which insight is retained. Examples include mild depression, obsessive compulsive disorder, and phobias.

neurotmesis: A lower motor neuron lesion.

neurotoxin: A poisonous or harmful chemical that attacks and damages nerve cells.

neurotransmitter: A chemical mediator that aids in the transmission of electrical impulses across the synapse. Examples include acetylcholine, norepinephrine, dopamine, and serotonin.

neurotrophic: Relating to the growth and nutrition of nervous tissue.

neutrophil: A white blood cell that ingests bacteria and thus helps fight infection; there are 2.0 to 7.5 x 109 neutrophils per liter of blood.

Niacin: Nicotinic acid; also known as vitamin B3; dietary sources include meat, peanut butter, and enriched cereals; the RDA for an adult is 18 mg/day; deficiencies lead to pellagra.

Noble's compression test: A special test of the knee used to assess IT band friction syndrome. *See* Special Tests-Knee (Appendix 16).

nociceptors: Afferent nerves responsible for sensing pain.

node: A small, rounded tissue mass.

node of Ranvier: The break or gap that occurs at the end of the Schwan cell in myelinated nerves.

nodule: A small lump caused by a group of cells or swelling of tissue that is usually abnormal.

nominal data: A type of nonparametric measure in which observations are classified according to a characteristic such as male or female, injured or not injured.

noninsulin-dependent diabetes: Also known as type II diabetes; a type of diabetes mellitus that occurs mainly in overweight adults over age 40 that can be treated with changes to the diet and the use of other drugs to increase natural production of insulin.

noninvasive: A medical procedure that does not involve penetration of the body; also used to refer to benign tumors that have remained localized.

nonnarcotic analgesic: A pharmacological agent that inhibits the release of neurotransmitters responsible for stimulating pain-sensing nerves and thus causes a relief of pain.

nonsteroidal anti-inflammatory drugs (NSAIDs): One of the many anti-inflammatory drugs that is not from the steroid family; used to reduce inflammation and pain. Examples include aspirin (acetylsalicylic acid), ibuprofen, naproxen sodium, piroxicam, and sulindac.

norepinephrine: A hormone secreted by the medulla responsible for the regulation of blood pressure.

normal force: The force directed perpendicular to a surface.

nosebleed: *See* epitaxis.

notch: An indentation in a bone.

nucleic acids: DNA or RNA present in the nucleus responsible for heredity.

nucleus: the DNA- and RNA-containing center of a cell.

nutrient: A substance required by the body to maintain its health, including carbohydrates, fats, proteins, minerals, and vitamins.

nystagmus: Involuntary lateral movement of the eyes.

Ober's test: A special test of the hip used to assess tensor fascia tightness. *See* Special Tests—Hip (Appendix 16).

obesity: A condition in which a person is more than 20% above the normal body weight for his or her age, height, and gender.

objective measure: A measurement technique that does not allow feelings or opinions (bias) of the investigator to affect the outcome; a test with precise scoring.

O'Brien test: A special test of the shoulder used to test for a slap lesion. *See* Special Tests—Shoulder (Appendix 16).

OBS: Abbreviation for "organic brain syndrome" or "observation."

obsessive-compulsive disorder: A tendency to perform repetitive behaviors to relieve anxiety, such as constantly washing the hands for fear of germs or repeatedly checking to see if the oven has been turned off or the door is locked; an unnatural concern that things are in order or in their exact place.

obturator nerve: The peripheral nerve from the lumbosacral plexus that innervates the hip adductors.

occlusion: To close; the state of being closed.

ocular: Of or pertaining to the eyes.

oculomotor nerve: Cranial nerve III responsible for voluntary motor control of the eyes. *See* Appendix 7.

ohm: A measure of the resistance to current flow.

olfactory nerve: Cranial nerve I responsible for the sense of smell. *See* Appendix 7.

one-tail (directional) test: A test for significance in which direction is predicted. It uses only one tail of the normal curve.

oocyte: A not quite fully developed egg cell; also called ovocyte. *See* primary and secondary oocyte.

oophorectomy: The surgical removal of an ovary.

open (kinetic) chain: An exercise in which the distal end is free to move. Example: knee extension or hamstring curls.

open (loose) packed position: A joint position when the bone ends in a position of least congruency. In this position, the joint will exhibit the most laxity.

ophthalmia: Inflammation of the eye, usually involving deeper structures; a severe conjunctivitis.

ophthalmologist: A physician specializing in ophthalmology.

ophthalmology: A medical specialty concerned with diseases and injuries of the eye.

Oppenheim's reflex: A reflex test in which the examiner runs a fingernail along the anterior tibia. A positive test is indicated by a positive Babinski's sign. *See also* Babinski's reflex/sign.

opposition: Movement of the thumb, toward the palm of the hand.

ophthalmic nerve: A small branch of the trigeminal nerve.

optic nerve: Cranial nerve II responsible for controlling the visual acuity. *See* Appendix 7.

optic neuritis: Inflammation of the optic nerve; often results in some vision loss.

optic: Relating to the eye.

optician: A specialist who makes and fits ophthalmic lenses.

ordinal data: Ordinal scale.

origin: The muscular attachment on the fixed segment.

orthotic: Orthosis; an external device used to correct or control biomechanics by limiting movement, providing support, increasing velocity or power, or generally enhancing function.

os: Bone; mouth-like.

os trigonum: The posterior process of the talus that serves as a site of attachment for the posterior talofibular ligament; it sometimes becomes separated from the talus to form this small triangular bone.

Osgood-Schlatter disease/syndrome: An apophysitis of the tibial tubercle caused by excessive repeated strain and seen most often in adolescents.

osmosis: The process of the passage of substances through a semi permeable membrane from an area of lesser concentration to an area of higher concentration.

ossification: The formation or maintenance of bone.

osteitis deformans: Paget's disease; a progressive disorder of abnormal bone growth resulting in a thickening and softening of bones.

osteitis: Inflammation of the bone.

osteoarthritis: A form of degenerative arthritis affecting joint cartilage and, subsequently, the underlying bone.

osteoblast: A cell responsible for bone formation.

osteochondritis dissecans: Degeneration within a joint in which there are small fragments of bone and cartilage in the joint causing pain, swelling, and loss of range of motion.

osteochondroma: A benign bone and cartilage tumor.

osteoclast: A cell responsible for breaking down unwanted bony tissue; a medical device used to correct bony deformity by fracturing the bone.

osteoma: A benign tumor of the bone.

osteomalacia: Softening of bones and loss of minerals due to vitamin D deficiency (also known as rickets in children).

osteomyelitis: Bacterial-induced inflammation affecting both bone and bone marrow.

osteonecrosis: Death of bone tissue.

osteophyte: A bony outgrowth near a joint, related to cartilage degeneration.

osteoporosis: A condition in which there is loss of bone tissue causing bones to become brittle and less dense leading to fractures.

otitis externa: Known as "swimmer's ear"; inflammation of the outer ear due to an infection.

otitis media: Inflammation of the middle ear often caused by nose and throat infection.

outcome measure: A means of assessment by evaluating the success of the treatment or program.

outward rotation: A rotation movement so as to turn the anterior aspect of the segment toward the outside or laterally; lateral rotation; external rotation.

ovaries: Bilateral glands at the opening of the fallopian tubes of the uterus responsible for production of eggs and the hormones estrogen and progesterone.

overpressure: A technique of applying pressure to a joint at its end range of motion to assess the end feel. *See* End Feel (Appendix 15).

over-the-counter: Pertaining to a medication that can be purchased without a physician's prescription.

overuse syndrome: A chronic injury caused by repetitive stress. Examples of overuse syndromes include tennis elbow, medial tibial stress syndrome, little league elbow, carpal tunnel syndrome, Osgood Schlatters, and pronator teres syndrome.

ovulation: Release of an ovum, usually occurring around mid-cycle.

ovum: Egg cell.

pacemaker: A small electronic device surgically implanted to produce and maintain a normal heart rhythm.

Paget's disease: A metabolic bone disorder occurring in the middle-aged and elderly in which bone does not form properly, causing bone weakening, thickening, and deformity; osteitis deformans.

pain scale: A scale used to assess the relative pain of an individual. One example shown below is the visual analog scale consisting of a 10-cm line with the descriptors on either end. Another example is a numeric pain scale ranging from 1 (no pain) to 10 (worst pain imaginable).

visual analog scale

no pain   worst pain imaginable

painful arc test: A special test of the shoulder in which the examiner notes the portion of the range of motion in which the patient exhibits pain.

palate: The roof of the mouth.

pallor: Pale skin, especially the face.

palpate: The act of using the hands or fingertips to discriminate tissue tension; to assess swelling, temperature, and to determine if point tenderness is present.

palpitation: An abnormally rapid and strong heartbeat.

palsy: Paralysis.

pancreas: A gland located behind the stomach in the upper left quadrant responsible for the production of enzymes that help to break down food and hormones; responsible for the regulation of glucose levels by the release of insulin and glucagons.

pancreatitis: Inflammation of the pancreas, often caused by alcoholism.

panic disorder: An emotional disorder characterized by anxiety attacks, often brought about by stress.

pap smear: A medical procedure in which epithelial cells are scraped from the cervix for examination to detect abnormal changes.

papilloma: A tumor, usually benign, found on skin and mucous membranes.

para: Beside, next to; abbreviation for "paraplegia."

paraffin bath: The use of melted paraffin wax as a thermo-therapeutic modality.

paralysis: Muscle weakness or an inability to contract a muscle or group of muscles including increased tone (spasticity) and decreased tone (flaccidity).

paramedical: Relating to the professions of individuals who have special training to provide various medical care but do not have a medical degree. Examples include nurses, physical therapists, athletic trainers, and emergency medical technicians.

paranoia: A psychosis characterized by unfounded suspicions of others.

paraplegia: Partial or complete loss of motor and sensory function of the legs.

parasite: An organism that inhabits and obtains its nutrients from another organism.

parasympathetic nervous system: The part of the autonomic nervous system that frequently opposes the sympathetic nervous system functioning mainly during relaxation.

parathyroid glands: Two pairs of small glands found in or near the thyroid that are stimulated to release parathyroid hormone by reductions of calcium in the blood.

parathyroid hormone: A hormone released by the parathyroid glands that controls the level of calcium in the blood.

parathyroidectomy: The surgical removal of a parathyroid gland.

parenteral: A substance administered by any route other than the through the mouth.

paresis: Loss of muscle strength; partial paralysis.

paresthesia: Tingling sensation; "pins and needles," loss of normal sensation.

Parkinson's disease: A disease of the basal ganglia. Symptoms include tremor and rigidity beginning in one arm and eventually affecting all limbs; caused by a lack of the chemical mediator dopamine.

paronychia: Bacterial or fungal infection, most commonly staphylococci or streptococci, causing inflammation around the nail beds.

passive range or motion (PROM): Range of motion performed by the examiner; the patient should remain relaxed. PROM is used to assess inert tissue.

passive stretch: A stretch to improve range of motion in which no active muscular contraction takes place.

patella: Kneecap.

patella alta: An abnormally high position of the patella in its groove.

patella baja: An abnormally low position of the patella in its groove.

pathogen: The microorganism or bacteria that causes disease.

pathogenesis: The process of the development of a disease or disorder.

pathology: The study of disease processes in order to understand the cause.

Patrick's test: *See* FABRE.

PDR (Physician's Desk Reference): A reference text for prescription drugs, published annually.

peak flow measurement: A method used to determine the maximum velocity that air is exhaled from a patient's lungs; used to diagnose lung conditions or to determine the effectiveness of medications to treat the condition.

Pearson r: A statistical measure of the correlation between two sets of parametric data.

peer review: An assessment of a body of work by a colleague with equal status.

pellagra: Vitamin B3 (niacin) deficiency causing dermatitis, diarrhea, and depression.

pelvic inflammatory disease (PID): The result of a bacterial infection, it is an inflammation of the reproductive organs in females; the use of tampons is linked to PID.

pepsin: The enzyme that helps digest protein.

peptic ulcer: A break or erosion of the mucosa caused by abnormally high concentrations of pepsin and acid.

perceived exertion: A measure used to assess an individual's perception of his/her exertion. *See* rating of perceived exertion and Borg scale.

perceptual motor skill: An activity that relies on special orientation, ocular control, and perception of body position in relation to the environment.

percussion: A diagnostic technique which involves tapping the surface to determine density of an area.

percutaneous: Through the skin.

perforation: The creation of a hole in an organ or body tissue caused by disease or injury.

periaqueductal grey (PAG): a midbrain structure important in the central biasing pain control theory in which descending impulses are initiated which travel down the dorsal horn to inhibit synaptic transmission of pain.

pericarditis: Inflammation of the membrane that surrounds the heart, causing chest pain and fever.

periosteum: The outer covering of bone.

periostitis: Inflammation of the periosteum.

peripheral nervous system: The nervous system outside of the central nervous system including the cranial nerves, spinal nerves, and all of its roots.

peripheral vascular disease: Reduced blood flow to the extremities due to a narrowing of the blood vessels, leading to pain and tissue damage in which necrosis may ensue.

peristalsis: A wave-like movement characteristic of tube-like structures for the purpose of moving material within the tube. The muscles immediately behind a material contract, and the ones immediately in front of a material relax.

peritoneum: The serous membrane that lines the abdomen.

peritonitis: Inflammation of the peritoneum.

pernicious: Describes serious diseases that are likely to result in death if untreated.

peroneal: Relating to the lateral (fibular) aspect of the lower leg.

peroneal nerve, common: One of the branches from the sciatic nerve; wraps around the fibular head before further dividing into the deep and superficial peroneal nerves; **deep**—found in the anterior compartment, innervates the tibialis anterior, the extensor hallicus longus, extensor digitorum, and the peroneus tertius; **superficial**—found in the lateral compartment, innervates peroneus longus and brevis.

peroneus: One of the lateral muscles of the lower leg. The peroneus longus and brevis cross the ankle posterior to the lateral malleolus and thus are responsible for plantar flexion and eversion of the ankle. The peroneus tertius lies just anterior to the lateral malleolus as it crosses the ankle and is thus responsible for dorsiflexion and eversion. The p. longus and brevis are innervated by the surperficial peroneal nerve while the p. tertius is innervated by the deep peroneal nerve.

Perthes' disease: *See* Legg-Calvé-Perthes disease.

pes: Foot.

pes anserine: Literally "foot of a bird"; the insertion of the semitendinosis, sartorius, and gracilis to the anteromedial tibia.

pes cavus: Abnormally high arches.

pes planus: Flat feet.

petit mal: A type of seizure characterized by a brief loss of awareness with no loss of consciousness.

petrissage: A type of therapeutic massage involving a kneading type of motion.

pH: A measure of the concentration of hydrogen in a solution; a pH less than 7 indicates an acidic solution and above 7 indicates an alkaline solution.

phagocyte: A cell that plays an important role in the healing process by digesting debris, microorganisms, and other unwanted material.

phalanges: The small bones of the fingers and toes.

Phalen's test: A special test of the wrist and hand to assess carpal tunnel syndrome. *See* Special Tests—Hand/Wrist (Appendix 16).

phantom limb: A sensation after a limb has been amputated that the limb still exists.

pharmacology: The study of the properties and actions of drugs.

pharyngitis: Inflammation of the pharynx, accompanied by sore throat, swollen glands, fever, and earache.

pharynx: The throat; a hollow tube that acts as the food and air passageway from the mouth and nose to the esophagus and larynx.

phases: In therapeutic modalities, a portion of a wave, or pulse. A pulse consisting of one phase is termed monophasic; two phases, biphasic; and more than two phases is termed polyphasic.

phenylketonuria: A hereditary disorder in which the individual cannot convert the amino acid phenylalanine and therefore it must not be consumed.

phlebitis: Inflammation of a vein.

phlebothrombosis: A blood clot in a vein.

phlegm: Sputum.

phobia: An unfounded fear of an event or situation. Phobias can have a profound effect on one's life because of the strong desire to avoid these situations.

phonophoresis: The use of ultrasound to deliver medication to deeper tissues.

photophobia: Oversensitivity of the eyes to light.

photosensitivity: An abnormal sensitivity to sunlight that results in skin irritation and rash.

phototherapy: An intervention with some form of light.

physically active: Defined by the NATA as individuals engaged in athletic, recreational, or occupational activities that require physical skills and utilize strength, power, endurance, speed, flexibility, range of motion, or agility.

physical activity: Defined by the NATA as athletic, recreational, or occupational activities that require physical skills and utilize strength, power, endurance, speed, flexibility, range of motion, or agility.

physical therapy: The treatment of injuries or disorders using mechanical treatments, including exercise, massage, manual therapies, mobilization, or the application of therapeutic modalities.

physiological motion: The voluntary motions such as flexion, extension, abduction, adduction, etc. Physiological motions require accessory motions.

physiology: The study of the functioning of living organisms.

piezoelectric effect: The vibration of the crystal in an ultrasound head when electrical current passes through it.

pinch test: A special test of the wrist and hand to assess the median nerve or carpal tunnel syndrome. *See* Special Tests—Hand/Wrist (Appendix 16).

pinched nerve: *See* neurapraxia.

pinkeye: *See* conjunctivitis.

PIP: Abbreviation for proximal interphalangeal joint.

piriformis syndrome: The compression of the sciatic nerve from the piriformis muscle caused by inflammation or hypertrophy. In some individuals the sciatic nerve pierces the piriformis muscle.

pitting edema: A thick viscous type of swelling associated with lymphedema that leaves an indentation (or "pit") when the skin is depressed during palpation.

pityriasis: Skin disease characterized by bran-like scales. Pityriasis alba is very common in children or adolescents and is characterized by pale macules on the face. Pityriasis rosea is a mild skin condition occurring in adults in which flat, scaly macules occur on the trunk and upper arms.

pivot shift test: A special test of the knee to assess the anterior cruciate ligament (ACL). *See* Special Tests—Knee (Appendix 16).

PKU: *See* phenylketonuria.

placebo: A sham treatment or chemically inactive substance given to a subject in a clinical trial. A placebo effect is the positive or negative response to the treatment due to the expectations of the treatment rather than the treatment itself.

planes of motion: *See* cardinal planes.

plantar fascia: A strong fibrous connective tissue on the plantar surface of the foot that runs from the medial tubercle of the calcaneus to the proximal metatarsal heads.

plantar wart: A wart on the sole of the foot, frequently painful and covered by callus.

plethysmography: A measurement technique for limb volume due to changes in blood pressure.

plexus: A network of nerves or blood vessels.

plica: A fold in the synovial tissue. A plica in the knee is a common site of pain.

plyometric: A type of exercise in which a quick stretch (or lengthening) is used just prior to the forceful contraction.

PMS: *See* premenstrual syndrome.

pneumonitis: Inflammation of the lungs.

pneumothorax: A condition in which air enters the pleural cavity causing chest pain and shortness of breath.

point tenderness: The pain that is produced when an area is palpated.

poliomyelitis: Commonly referred to as polio; an infectious viral disease of the motor cells of the spinal cord.

pollex: The thumb.

polycystic kidney disease: Multiple cysts on the kidneys.

polycystic ovary syndrome: Multiple cysts on the ovaries.

polycythemia: Excessive hemoglobin concentration.

polydipsia: Excessive thirst.

polymyalgia rheumatica: A rare disease affecting older adults resulting in generalized pain and stiffness in the hips, thighs, shoulders, and neck.

polyneuritis: Inflammation of multiple nerves.

polyp: A tumor projecting from a mucous membrane that can become cancerous.

polyuria: Excessive production of urine, a common sign of diabetes mellitus and other diseases.

post-concussion syndrome: Symptoms following a mild head injury that can include headaches, dizziness, mild mental impairment (difficulty concentrating), and fatigue lasting a few months to an indefinite period of time.

posterior draw (drawer) sign: A special test of the knee to assess the posterior cruciate ligament (PCL). *See* Special Tests—Knee (Appendix 16).

post-traumatic stress disorder (PTSD): A condition following a frightening or stressful life event in which the individual suffers from recurring dreams, difficulty sleeping, "flashbacks," and fear of reoccurance of the event.

postural sway: A measure of balance, generally a measure of the time and distance excursion from one's center of balance.

posture: The attitude of the body; the position maintained by the body in standing or in sitting; the alignment and positioning of the body in relation to gravity, center of mass, and base of support; the position of the body or body part in relation to space and/or to other body parts. Functionally, the anticipation about, in response to, displacement of the body's center of mass. (*Quick Reference Dictionary for Physical Therapy*, 2000).

Pott's fracture: A fracture of the distal fibula and medial malleolus of the tibia with an outward displacement of the foot.

power: The amount of work performed per unit of time. $p = (w \times d)/time$.

predictor: A variable used to predict behavior.

premenopausal: The period that accounts for the years leading up to menopause.

premenstrual syndrome: The physical and emotional symptoms that occur 7 to 14 days prior to menstruation or from ovulation to the onset of menstruation; symptoms include depression, irritability, abdominal pain, and fatigue.

presbyopia: Also known as far-sighted; the degradation of near vision occurring naturally with age due to a loss of elasticity of the lens of the eyes, generally resulting in the need for reading glasses.

pressure: The ratio of force to the area where the force is applied.

pressure point (trigger point): A tender point that has a relationship to an area of pain.

primary oocyte: The ovum at the end of maturation but before the first division of meiosis.

prime mover: A muscle primarily responsible for a given movement; example: the biceps brachii muscle is a prime mover for elbow flexion.

profile test: A special test for posterior cruciate ligament instability. Also called Sag test. *See* Special Tests—Knee (Appendix 16).

prognosis: An assessment of the probable outcome of the patient's disease.

progressive resistance exercise (PRE): Developed by Delorme, it is an exercise method consisting of the use of weights lifted through a range of motion against gravity. The amount of weight and the number of repetitions is progressively increased as follows: First set, 10 reps at 50% of 10 repetitions maximum (RM); second set, 10 reps at 75% of 10 RM; third set at 100% of 10 RM.

The Oxford technique is the same except the percentages are performed in reverse order. *See also* DAPRE.

prolapse: Disc herniation of the nucleus pulposus through the annulus fibrosis.

pronation: The act of turning downward; in the foot, pronation is dependent upon whether the motion is performed open or closed chain. During closed chain movement, pronation involves plantar flexion, eversion, and adduction. During open chain movement, pronation involves dorsiflexion, eversion, and abduction.

pronator teres syndrome: A compression of the median nerve by the pronator teres muscle.

prophylactic: Preventative measure.

proprioception: A sense or awareness of position.

proprioceptive neuromuscular facilitation (PNF): A method of using passive, active, and active-assisted range of motion to improve flexibility and neuromuscular strength. There are many techniques of PNF.

proprioceptor: A receptor that responds to changes in the body such as movement and position.

prostate gland: An accessory gland located under the bladder and vas deferens in men. It is responsible for the production of part of the semen. It can become enlarged in older men, impairing urination and subsequently causing damage to the kidneys.

prosthesis: A device used to improve function and/or to replace a missing or impaired organ or body part.

proteinemia: Excess protein in the blood.

proteinuria: Protein in the urine.

protraction: Abduction of the scapula.

protusion: The least severe disc herniation in which the nucleus pulposus does not actually exit through the annulus fibrosis, rather a "bulge" puts pressure on the nerve root.

proximal: A term of description denoting a segment or body part that is nearer the central point (or core); closer to the point of origin.

pruritus: Itching.

psoriasis: A chronic skin disorder characterized by itchy, scaly, red patches most commonly found on the elbows, knees, forearms, legs, and scalp.

psoriatic arthritis: A type of arthritis caused by psoriasis.

psychogenic: Caused by or related to psychological/emotional disorders.

psychological: Relating to behavior or the processes of the mind.

psychosis: A severe mental disorder in which there is a loss of reality and an inability to think clearly.

psychosomatic: Describes physical signs and symptoms that are influenced by psychological factors.

psychotherapy: Medical treatment of emotional disorders.

Ptosis: Drooping of the upper eyelid.

pulmonary: Referring to or associated with the lungs.

pulp: A soft tissue mass such as the pads of the fingers; the soft tissue inside a tooth containing blood vessels and nerves.

pulsed current: Regular intervals of electrical currents that are packaged into groups of three or more pulses.

pulsed ultrasound: The use of ultrasound in which there are intermittent on and off cycles so as to reduce the thermal effects.

pupil: The portion of the iris that controls the amount of light that enters the eye by constricting or dilating.

purpura: Small hemorrhages causing purplish spots on the skin.

purulent: Pus-containing infection.

pus: A thick, yellowish fluid containing bacteria and necrotic white blood cells.

pustule: A small blister containing pus.

pyelolithotomy: Surgical removal of a kidney stone.

pyelonephritis: A bacterial infection causing inflammation of the kidney.

pyloric sphincter: The circular muscle between the stomach and small intestine that controls the passage of food.

quadriplegia: Partial or complete loss of motor and sensory function of all four limbs.

qualitative research: An approach to measurement that is more subjective or judgmental.

quantitative research: An approach to measurement that is more objective.

quinapril (Accupril): An ACE inhibitor.

R

radial nerve: One of the terminal branches of the brachial plexus arising from the nerve roots C5-T1. The radial nerve passes posteriorly and supplies the sensation and innervates the muscles of the posterior upper arm and arm.

radiating pain: Pain that emanates from a pathology and often follows the path of a nerve.

radiation: Energy traveling in the form of waves; a method of electromagnetic (including heat) transfer in which no medium is required.

radiation therapy: A radioactive treatment for diseases such as cancer that attacks the targeted tissue cells.

radical mastectomy: A treatment for breast cancer in which the entire breast, pectoral muscles, lymph nodes, and other tissues are removed.

radical surgery: Extreme or drastic measures, often a final resort; the surgical removal of tissue affected by disease.

radiculitis: *See* radiculopathy.

radiculopathy: Disorder of the spinal nerve root; radiating pain that follows a nerve distribution.

radiography (x-ray): A diagnostic procedure in which images of the inside of the body are formed using a form of radiation that is projected through the body and onto film.

radius: One of the long bones of the arm, it is the bone located on the thumb side. When the arm is in anatomical position, it sits lateral to the ulna.

ramipril (Altrace): An ACE inhibitor.

random access memory (RAM): The primary memory of a computer.

randomization: The selection of sample groups in which each member of the population has equal opportunity of being selected.

range of motion (ROM): The motion available at a joint in each plane, measured in degrees.

rapid eye movement (REM): The stage of deep sleep in which the eyes are moving.

rate of rise: Related to the shape of a waveform. It is a measure of how quickly the impulse rises from 0 to peak amplitude.

rating of perceived exertion (RPE): *See* Borg scale.

ratio scales: A measurement scale based on order in which there are equal units between measures and a base of zero. Examples include force, distance, number of repetitions, and time.

Raynaud's disease: A condition of unknown cause in which there is a vasospasm of the blood vessels supplying the fingers and toes causing them to become pale, numb, and painful when exposed to cold.

reaction time: The period of time from stimulus to reaction.

receptive field: An area supplied by a given nerve.

receptor: A sensory nerve ending; nerve cell that responds to a stimulus; specialized sensory cells that detect chemical, mechanical, thermal and other changes; see also mechanoreceptor, proprioceptor.

reciprocal inhibition: A reflex relaxation of the antagonist muscle group upon agonist contraction.

rectilinear: The path of movement along a straight line.

rectum: The distal end of the large intestine connecting the large intestine to the anus.

rectus femoris tightness test: *See* Kendall test.

reduction of fracture: A procedure to realign the ends of a fracture: may be performed closed (no surgery) or open (surgical procedure).

referred pain: Pain in an area other than the site of injury or illness. Example: Kerr's sign is pain in the left shoulder caused by injury or illness to the spleen.

reflex: An involuntary activity involving simple circuitry from which a stimulus causes an automatic reaction such as the automatic withdrawal of the hand from a source of heat. *See also* deep tendon reflex.

reflex sympathetic dystrophy (RSD): Pain disproportionate or delayed recovery not consistent with the severity of injury. Signs and symptoms include hypersensitivity, decreased strength, spasm, edema, and dermatologic changes.

regeneration: The process of repair, regrowth, or restoration of a tissue following injury.

rehydration: A process of restoring the normal water, sodium, glucose, and electrolyte levels of the body.

Reiter's syndrome: A common reactive arthritic condition; an inflammation disorder affecting one or more joints, the urethra, and sometimes the conjunctiva.

relapse: The return of symptoms following a period of improvement.

relative refractory period: The period following depolarization when the membrane is "repolarizing," in which an action potential could occur if stimulus of sufficient strength (greater than that required to reach threshold when at rest) is applied.

reliability: A measure of the consistency of the data.

relocation test: A test for shoulder anterior apprehension in which the examiner applies a posterior force to the apprehensive patient during the anterior apprehension test. A reduction in apprehension is a positive sign.

REM: *See* rapid eye movement.

remission: The period of time in which there is a disappearance of a disease or its symptoms.

renal: Nephric; referring to the kidney.

renal cell carcinoma: A common type of kidney cancer.

renal colic: Severe pain in a kidney caused by a kidney stone.

repetitive strain injury: An injury that occurs when the same movement is repeated continuously. Common repetitive strain injuries include carpal tunnel syndrome and medial tibial stress syndrome.

residual: Something that lingers or remains; a permanent condition that results from an injury or illness.

residual volume: The air that remains in the lungs after a forcible exhalation (approximately 60 to 100 cubic inches).

resistance: A force applied against another force; the opposition to the flow of electrical current, measured in ohms; electrical impedance.

resistive force: A force that resists the motion caused by a motive force. When lifting a weight against gravity, the muscles provide the motive force while gravity provides a resistive force. When lowering a weight with gravity, gravity provides the motive force, while the muscles provide a resistive force.

respiratory arrest: The absence of breathing.

respiratory distress syndrome: A life-threatening condition in which an individual is unable to breath normally caused by injury or illness leading to a decrease in oxygen to the tissues.

respiratory failure: An increase in carbon dioxide and decrease in oxygen in the blood caused by the failure of the body to adequately exchange gases.

resting pulse: The normal pulse rate expected of an individual while at rest (80 bpm in adults).

retina: The light sensitive portion of the eye that contains the rods and cones.

retinaculum: A dense, fibrous retaining band that acts to hold tendons in place.

retinopathy: A disease of the retina most commonly a consequence of hypertension or diabetes mellitus.

retraction: Adduction of the scapula.

retro: Denoting backward or behind.

retrograde: Moving backward; retrograde amnesia is the inability to remember details prior to the onset of injury or illness.

retroversion: Of the hip, it refers to external rotation.

Reye's syndrome: A rare disorder mainly affecting children and teens, characterized by vomiting, disorientation, lethargy, and liver damage following a viral infection. May be linked to the use of aspirin in the treatment of viral infection.

rheo: Electrical current; blood flow.

rheobase: The minimum current required to reach tissue excitation when maximum phase duration is used.

rheumatoid arthritis: A chronic, systemic, inflammatory disease of the joints, particularly the fingers, wrists, feet, ankles, hips, knees and shoulders; can also affect other joints such as costovertebral, sternoclavicular etc. Diagnosed by the presence of rheumatoid factor in the blood.

rheumatoid factors: The presence of antibodies in individuals with rheumatoid arthritis (only 80% of individuals with rheumatoid arthritis test positive for rheumatoid factors).

rhinitis: Inflammation of the nasal passage causing congestion, sneezing, runny nose caused by the common cold or allergies (allergic rhinitis).

rickets: *See* osteomalacia.

right rotation: A rotation of the trunk or neck toward the right.

rigidity: In a muscle, resistance to movement throughout the range of motion; abdominal rigidity caused by muscle guarding is often a sign of internal bleeding and injury to an organ. **Decerebrate**—indicating brainstem injury; extension and adduction of the upper extremity joints; and extension, internal rotation, and plantar flexion in the lower extremity. **Decorticate**—Indicating injury above the brainstem, flexion and adduction of the upper extremity joints, extension, internal rotation and plantar flexion in the lower extremity.

ringworm: Tinea; a highly contagious fungal infection of the skin that can be spread by direct contact; appears as a red scaly circle; common in wrestling.

Rinne's test: A test that utilizes a tuning fork to determine if hearing loss is due to perception or conduction. The tuning fork is held in the air near the ear and then placed on the mastoid bone. If the sound is heard longer when the tuning fork is held in the air, the test is positive for perception loss. If the sound is heard longer when the tuning fork is in contact with the mastoid, the test is negative and indicates conduction loss.

RNA (ribonucleic acid): Found in all cells; concerned with protein synthesis.

Rocky mountain spotted fever: A rare disease transmitted to humans by ticks; signs and symptoms include fever, muscle pain, and a spreading red rash. Treated with antibiotics. Untreated, the disease may be fatal.

roentenogram: X-ray.

Rolfing: A type of therapeutic massage involving soft tissue manipulation with the intent of balancing the body within a gravitational field.

Romberg's sign: A test for neurological dysfunction in which the patient stands with eyes open and arms to the side. The patient then closes his or her eyes and the examiner notes disturbances in balance. Modified Romberg's sign is performed on a single limb to assess neuromuscular control and somatosensory input from the lower extremity (especially the foot).

Roo's test: A special test of the shoulder specifically for thoracic outlet syndrome. *See* Special Tests—Shoulder (Appendix 16).

rosacea: A skin disease affecting adults (usually 30 to 50 years old) characterized by chronic redness on the forehead, cheeks, chin, and nose caused by dilated blood vessels.

rotation: Motion that follows a circular path and takes place about an axis.

rotator cuff: A structure made up of the SITS (supraspinatus, infraspinatus, teres minor, subscapularis) muscles that in addition to rotation of the shoulder play an important role in the stability of the shoulder joint.

rubella: German measles; an acute, mild infection caused by the rubella virus. Signs and symptoms include rash and fever. Can cause birth defects when a woman is infected during the early stages of pregnancy.

runner's knee: *See* iliotibial band (ITB) friction syndrome.

rupture: A break or tear in a tissue.

sacral apex: A special test of the sacroiliac joint. *See* Special Tests—Hip (Appendix 16).

sacroiliac: The joint between the ilium of the pelvis and the sacrum.

sacroiliitis: Inflammation of the sacroiliac joints.

sacrum: The broad, spade-shaped bone located at the bottom of the spine forming the posterior wall of the pelvis. The sacrum is formed by the fusion of five sacral vertebrae.

SAD: *See* seasonal affective disorder.

sag test: *See* profile test.

saggital plane: Midsaggital; divides the body into left and right parts. Motions that take place in this plane include flexion/extension.

SAID principle: Abbreviation for "specific adaptation to imposed demands"; the body will adapt to whatever increased demands are placed on it; related to the overload principle.

saline: A solution that contains 0.9% sodium chloride.

sarcoidosis: Besnier-Boeck-Schaumann disease; a rare systemic disease of unknown cause consisting of inflammation and fibrosis especially of the lungs, but also in the lymph nodes, liver, skin, glands, and eyes.

sarcoma: A type of connective tissue cancer, usually highly malignant.

Saturday night palsy: Temporary paralysis of the arm after extended pressure on the nerves in the axilla. The name is derived from the situation when one "passes out" in a position where there will be pressure on the axilla (and the nerves in the brachial plexus) for an extended period of time. The axillary nerve or radial nerve is commonly affected, leading to the temporary inability to abduct the shoulder or extend the elbow.

scabies: A highly contagious skin disorder caused by mites. The female mite burrows into the skin producing an intensely itchy vesicular eruption.

scalenectomy: The surgical removal of one or more of the scalene muscles.

scaphoid: Navicular of the hand; the most lateral bone in the first (proximal) layer of carpals. A common site of nonunion in fractures due to poor blood supply.

scapula: The large, flat, triangular bone of the shoulder girdle that sits posterior and lateral over the ribs. The lateral angle of the scapula forms the glenoid fossa that articulates with the humerus, and just superior lies the acromion process that articulates with the clavicle.

scapulohumeral: Relating to the scapula and humerus. Scapulohumeral rhythm refers to the relationship of movement of the scapula to movement of the humerus.

Scheuermann's disease (juvenile kyphosis): An adolescent skeletal disease that results in a hunched back.

schizophrenia: A type of psychosis characterized by distorted perception, abnormal thought processes, and personality disorders, including split or multiple personalities.

sciatica: Pain along the sciatic nerve most commonly caused by nerve root compression or piriformis syndrome.

sclera: The tough, white portion of the eye.

scleroderma: A painful hardening and contraction of the connective tissues; can remain localized or may spread to other tissues; can result in death.

scoliosis: A congenital or acquired abnormal lateral deviation of the vertebral column, commonly "S" or "C" shaped.

screening: A process of evaluating an otherwise healthy person in order to detect potential abnormalities. Preseason or preparticipation screening is common prior to the start of an athletic season.

seasonal affective disorder (SAD): A psychological, emotional disorder characterized by depression brought on by the change of season (particularly fall and winter) and shorter days.

seborrhea: Excessive secretion of sebum (oil) on the face and scalp.

sebum: An oily secretion from the sebaceous glands.

second-class lever: Is a type of machine in which the resistive force is between the axis and motive forces. Examples include a wheel barrow and a nut cracker. Most eccentric actions in the body are performed by second class levers due to the force of gravity acting as the motive force during an eccentric contraction. The advantage of this type of lever arrangement is that the motive force always has a longer level arm and thus a greater force advantage in producing an equal torque.

second impact syndrome: A head injury, sometimes apparently very mild, that occurs before the symptoms of a previous head injury have resolved. This is a very serious injury with a mortality rate of 50%.

secondary cell death: Death of the cells due to lack of oxygen secondary to edema.

secondary: Not primary; describes a disease or injury caused by another one (primary).

secondary oocyte: The larger of two ovums following the first division of meiosis.

second order neuron: Afferent neurons in the spinal cord or brain.

sedatives: A pharmacologic agent that has a calming effect used to relieve anxiety, tension, and insomnia.

seizure: Sudden electrical hyperactivity in the brain, causing loss of consciousness or convulsions.

sepsis: Destruction of tissue by bacteria; can result in an infection in which bacteria is dangerously spread into the bloodstream.

septic arthritis: Inflammatory joint disease caused by a bacterial infection.

septicemia: Also known as blood poisoning; an invasion of microorganisms into the blood stream caused by infection often accompanied by abscess and toxemic symptoms.

septic shock: A severe and life-threatening consequence of sepsis in which blood pressure drops due to blood poisoning.

sequela: The result or consequence of a previous injury or disorder.

sequestration: A severe type of disk herniation in which the disk fragments into small pieces.

serotonin: A neurotransmitter important to sleep and chemical mediator thought to play a role in the inflammatory process.

sesamoid: Small round bone or cartilage in a tendon that acts to increase leverage by increasing the angle of pull of the tendon (eg, patella).

Sever's disease: Calcaneal apophysitis.

sharpened Romberg: A variation of the Romberg sign in which the patient stands with one foot directly in front of the other (heel to toe).

shear: The movement of one surface over another within the same plane of motion.

shin splints: A generic term for "shin pain" or medial tibial stress syndrome.

shingles: *See* herpes zoster.

shock: A result of circulatory collapse caused by severe bleeding, cardiac or respiratory distress, allergic reaction, pain, or emotional distress. Can become life-threatening without treatment.

shunt: A passageway (congenital or artificial) that channels or diverts blood from one area to another.

sickle cell anemia: A hereditary disease affecting African Americans in which red blood cells have a characteristic "sickling" (oblong shape). These cells cease to be circulated, causing anemia.

side effect: An unwanted consequence of a treatment.

sigmoidoscopy: The use of a scope to examine the rectum and the large intestine.

sign: A characteristic of a disease or injury that is observed by the examiner and may or may not have been noticed by the patient (compare to symptom).

sign of buttock: A special test for tumor or trochanteric bursitis. *See* Special Tests—Hip (Appendix 16).

significance: A statistical term that is used to describe a difference in mean scores or a relationship that is not due simply to chance.

silver fork fracture: A Colles' fracture in which the profile appears to take on the shape of a fork.

sinus rhythm: Normal heart rhythm.

sinusitis: Inflammation of the the sinuses, usually as a result of a bacterial infection.

sleep apnea: A condition in which there is a temporary cessation of breathing during sleep.

slipped capital femoral epiphysis: A posterior or inferior slippage of the femoral head seen most commonly in boys age 10 to 17.

slipped disk: *See* disk injury or prolapse.

slow twitch fiber: *See* type I fiber.

slump test: Special test for the presence of spinal cord, dura, or nerve root injury in which the patient is seated with one knee extended, the trunk flexed while the examiner passively flexes the neck.

Smith's fracture: A reverse Colles' fracture in which the displacement is toward the palmar side.

Snellen's chart: A chart used to assess visual acuity that has printed letters that decrease in size on each subsequent line.

solar plexus: The largest plexus in the body, located behind the stomach.

soma: Cell body.

somatic: Pertaining to the body.

spasm: An involuntary abnormal muscular contraction.

spastic paralysis: Spasticity or increased reflex activity with concomitant weakness of the limbs caused by disease of the corticospinal tract. *See also* spasticity.

spasticity: Muscle stiffness and resistance that gives way to increased passive movement. *See also* spastic paralysis.

speed's test: A special test of the shoulder to determine the presence of biceps tendonitis or biceps tendon subluxation. *See* Special Tests—Shoulder (Appendix 16).

spermatic cord torsion: An injury to the testicle, usually a direct blow, causing the testicles to revolve in the scrotum producing pain, nausea, vomiting, and inflammation, and can lead to atrophy. Physician referral is recommended.

sphygmomanometer: The measurement instrument used to assess blood pressure.

spica: A figure-8 type wrapping procedure around a joint.

spina bifida: A birth defect in which there is a failure of the spine to fuse, leaving the spine underdeveloped and exposed. There are various degrees of this deformity.

spina bifida occulta: The least severe form of spina bifida, in which there is no protrusion of the spinal cord or its membrane.

spinal fusion: A surgical procedure in which two or more adjacent vertebrae are joined using bone fragments or surgical hardware to treat spinal instability.

spine of the scapula: The nearly horizontal bone across the dorsum of the scapula above which sits the supraspinatus muscle and below which sits the infraspinatus muscle. The lateral end of the spine of the scapula forms the acromion process (point of the shoulder).

spirometer: A gasometer that measures respiratory gases; device to measure lung capacity by measuring the volume of air exhaled.

spleen: An organ located in the upper left quadrant of the abdomen whose function is to produce lymphocytes and store red blood cells.

splenectomy: Surgical removal of the spleen.

splint: A device that is used to immobilize a body part.

spondylitis: Inflammation of the synovial joints of the vertebrae.

spondylolisis: A defect in the pars interarticularis of the vertebra known as a "collared Scottie dog."

spondylolisthesis: A defect in the pars interarticularis of the vertebra with a forward slippage of the vertebral body known as a "decapitated Scottie dog."

SPORTDiscuss: A bibliographic database, international in scope, covering all aspects of sport, fitness, recreation, and related fields. Articles from more than 2000 sport-related journals, monographs, articles, books, theses, and CD-ROMs in English, French, and other languages are indexed for inclusion. The Sport Information Resource Center (SIRC), the database provider, is the largest resource center in the world collecting and disseminating information in the area of sport, physical education, physical fitness, and sports medicine.

sprain: To stretch or tear a ligament; the fibrous connective tissue that attaches bone to bone.

Spurling's test: Special test of the cervical spine for nerve root compression. *See* Special Tests—Spine (Appendix 16).

sputum: Saliva and mucus that is coughed up from the lungs and airway.

squish test: Special test of the sacroiliac joint. See Special Tests—Hip (Appendix 16).

standard deviation: A measure of how spread out the observed scores are from their mean.

standard error of the mean: The amount of error in the prediction of the true (population) mean.

standardized test: A test that has been developed and tested, has established procedures and norms, and demonstrated reliability and validity.

staphylococci: A gram-positive bacteria that causes skin infections and other purulent infections.

stasis: A slowing or blockage of the normal flow of fluid.

stenosis: Abnormal narrowing of a passage.

sternum: The long, flat bone central to the thorax articulating with the clavicle and the cartilage of the ribs, made up of the manubrium, body, and xiphoid process.

steroids: Fat soluble organic compounds naturally occurring or synthetic. The naturally occurring steroids include androgen, estrogen, progesterone, bile salts, and sterols. Synthetic steroids include corticosteroids and anabolic steroids. Corticosteroids include cortisone, hydrocortisone, and corticosterone, which have powerful anti-inflammatory effects, while aldosterone is used primarily for the regulation of sodium and water. Anabolic steroids include ethylestranol, methandienone, nandrolone, norethandrolone, oxymesterone, and stanalone. They have been linked to serious side effects including depression, hostility, suicide, liver damage, and other severe health disorders, and death.

stinger: *See* neurapraxia.

stoma: Mouth; an artificial opening created surgically.

strabismus: Abnormal alignment of the eyes, such as heterotropia when one eye looks upward and one downward, or crossed eyes.

strain: A stretch or tear in a muscle or tendon; the deformation of an object; *see also* stress-strain curve (expressed as units of force x length or joules).

strength: A measure of a muscle's ability to exert a maximal force against a resistance.

strength-duration curve: A graphical illustration of the relationship between the duration of an electrical current and the strength (intensity) of the current needed to reach an action potential. As the duration is increased, less intensity is required to achieve the same result.

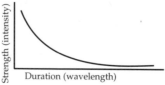

strep throat: Streptococcus bacteria causing sore throat, fever, and swollen lymph nodes.

streptococci: Gram-positive bacteria that cause a variety of diseases including scarlet fever, pneumonia, and strep throat.

stress: An internal force divided by the area over which it is applied. Expressed in Newtons/m^2 or pascals.

stress fracture: Also called fatigue fracture; a fracture caused by repetitive motions such as running, marching, etc.

stress-strain curve: A plot of the relationship of stress to strain (the elastic modulus) of a material.

stretch-shortening exercise: *See* plyometric.

stroke: Apoplexy; a sudden interruption of blood flow to the brain causing loss of consciousness, sensation, and movement. Damage to the brain due to lack of blood supply (from blockage in an artery) or rupture of a blood vessel leads to complete or partial loss of function in the area of the body that is controlled by that portion of the brain. Severity varies greatly.

stye: Bacterial infection causing inflammation in the follicle of an eyelash.

subacute: Condition that appears just beyond and is less severe than the acute stage.

subcutaneous: Below the cutaneous layer (skin).

subdural hematoma: Bleeding in the brain below the dura matter, usually venous bleeding with slower onset of symptoms (could be as long as 24 hours to 1 month). Compare to epidural hematoma.

subjective measure: A measure based on judgment of an individual (contrast to objective).

subluxation: A partial or incomplete dislocation, or a dislocation followed by an immediate and spontaneous relocation.

substance P: A neurotransmitter thought to play an important role in initiation of transmission of an impulse along a first order neuron and at the synapse between first order and second order neurons.

substantia gelatinosa: An area in the dorsal horn of the spinal cord thought to play an important role in the control of pain. *See also* gate control theory.

substitution: The improper use of other muscles to perform an activity. The use of substitute motions can promote incorrect motor programming and dysfunction.

subtalar: Below the talus; the articulation between the talus and calcaneus.

sudden infant death syndrome (SIDS): The unexpected death of an otherwise healthy baby; the cause is unknown.

sulcus sign: A special test of the shoulder to assess glenohumeral instability. *See* Special Tests—Shoulder (Appendix 16).

superior: Above.

supination: The act of turning upward; in the foot, supination is dependent upon whether the motion is performed open or closed chain. During closed chain movement, supination involves dorsiflexion, inversion, and abduction. During open chain movement, supination involves plantar flexion, inversion, and adduction.

suprascapular nerve: The nerve supplying the supraspinatus and infraspinatus.

sural: Relating to the leg (lower leg).

suture: Surgical closure of a wound; an immovable joint such as the sutures of the skull.

sway index: An indirect measure of balance or postural sway, it is the standard deviation of time and distance the individual spent away from his or her center of balance. The Chattecx Dynamic Balance System (Chattanooga Group Inc) uses the sway index.

swimmer's ear: *See* otitis externa.

swing phase: The phase during a walking cycle between toe off and heel strike.

symmetrical: The same; similar bilaterally.

symptom (Sx): A characteristic of a disease or injury that is experienced and described by the patient (compare to sign).

synapse: The act of an electrical nerve impulse crossing from one neuron to the next; the gap between two neurons (synaptic cleft).

syncope: Fainting, loss of consciousness due to insufficient blood flow to the brain.

syndrome: A group of signs and symptoms that when found together are characteristics of a particular disorder.

synergist: A muscle that "assists" an agonist; a drug interaction that together produces a desired effect that each drug would not produce if given alone.

synovectomy: Surgical removal of a synovial membrane.

synovial fluid: A viscous fluid secreted by the synovial membrane found in synovial joints, tendon sheaths, and bursa.

synovial membrane: The thin mesothelium and connective tissue membrane that encloses a moveable joint and secretes synovial fluid.

synovitus: Inflammation of the synovial membrane. Signs and symptoms include redness, swelling, joint stiffness, and pain. Common causes are rheumatoid arthritis or infection.

synthesis: The union of chemical elements so as to form a whole.

systemic: Affecting the whole body.

systemic lupus erythematosus: An autoimmune inflammatory connective tissue disease of unknown cause in which fever, rash, arthritis, anemia, and hemorrhages in the skin and mucous membranes occur. In more serious cases, inflammation of the pericardium and damage to the kidneys and central nervous system can occur.

systolic pressure: Blood pressure measured while the heart is contracting; the normal systolic pressure in an adult is 120 mmHg, normal diastolic pressure is 80 mmHg, recorded as 120/80 mmHg.

T cell: *See* T-lymphocyte.

tachycardia: A fast heart rate, usually over 100 beats per minute in adults.

talar tilt: A special test of the ankle to assess the medial and lateral ligaments. *See* Special Tests—Foot/Ankle (Appendix 16).

talipes equinovarus: Clubfoot; weightbearing occurs on the ball of the foot and lateral aspect of the foot.

tapotement: A massage technique involving percussion of "cupped" hands.

tarsal tunnel syndrome: Tibial nerve compression as it crosses the ankle medially deep to the flexor retinaculum and tibiocalcaneal ligament through the tarsal tunnel.

temporomandibular joint syndrome (TMJ): A disorder of the temporomandibular joint causing headache and tenderness of the jaw and teeth.

tendinitis: Inflammation of the tendon.

tendon: A strong, fibrous connective tissue that connects muscle to bone.

tendon transfer: The repositioning of a tendon for the purpose of redefining the role of the muscle and/or tendon.

tennis elbow: *See* lateral epicondylitis.

tenosynovitis: Inflammation of the synovial sheath of a tendon.

tensile: Referring to tension.

tensiometer: A device designed to measure the amount of tension or force applied.

testicular torsion: Severe pain and swelling of a testicle due to twisting of the spermatic cord.

testosterone: A male sex hormone produced in the testes in males and in the adrenal cortex in males and females; responsible for the development of male secondary sex characteristics.

tetanus: A sometimes fatal disease characterized by painful tonic muscular contractions caused by bacteria present in soil and manure. The DTaP vaccine is given at 2, 4, 6, 15 months, and 4 to 6 years. Persons receiving all five doses may not require booster until age 50. Most adults have not, and thus should receive a booster every 10 years.

tetracycline: One of the antibiotic drugs used to treat a variety of infections.

thoracodorsal nerve: The nerve supplying the latissimus dorsi, it arises from C6-8 and the posterior trunk of the brachial plexus.

thenar: The thumb side of the "heel of the hand."

therapeutic range: The range of dosage of a treatment modality of drug that will produce the desired effects without the unwanted side effects.

thermotherapy: A therapeutic modality involving the use of heat.

third-class lever: A type of machine in which the motive force is between the axis and resistive forces. Examples include a snow shovel, an oar, and a baseball bat. In the body, most joint movements are performed by third-class levers. The advantage of a third-class lever is speed of movement and range of motion. A distinct disadvantage is that the motive force will always have a shorter lever arm, thus requiring greater amount of force to produce the same amount of torque.

third-order neuron: Afferent neurons in the brain.

Thomas test: A special test of the hip to assess hip flexion contracture. *See* Special Tests—Hip (Appendix 16).

Thompson's test: A special test of the Achille's tendon to assess for rupture. *See* Special Tests—Foot/Ankle (Appendix 16).

thoracic outlet syndrome (TOS): A condition in which the brachial plexus and/or subclavian artery become stretched or more likely, impinged, causing radiating pain, numbness (neurogenic symptoms), and reduced circulation (vascular symptoms). Common causes are scalene muscles, cervical rib anomaly, depressed shoulder, and poor posture. In over 90% of the cases, there are no vascular symptoms.

thorax: The chest.

threshold: The point above which a reaction will take place and below which no reaction will occur. Threshold must be met in order to reach an action potential. Once threshold is met, there is complete depolarization (all or none response).

thrombectomy: Removal of a blood clot.

thrombocytopenic purpura: An abnormally small number of platelets in the blood, causing abnormal bruising due to bleeding.

thromboembolism: An obstruction caused by a thrombus (clot) that has dislodged and traveled from another area.

thrombophlebitis: Inflammation of a vein with concomitant clot formation in the affected area.

thrombosis: The formation of a blood clot within a vessel.

thrombus: A blood clot.

thyroid gland: A gland located posterior and lateral to the larynx responsible for the secretion of thyroid hormone and calcitonin.

thyroiditis: Inflammation of the thyroid gland.

tibia: The large weightbearing bone of the lower leg.

tibial nerve: One of the branches of the sciatic nerve that extends posterior along the back of the leg below the knee and supplies the muscles of the posterior leg.

tibial torsion: Excessive rotation of the tibia.

Tietze's syndrome: A painful condition in which there is inflammation of the costocartilage.

tinea corporis: An infection on the body area caused by a fungus.

tinea cruris: Also known as jock itch; an infection in the groin area caused by a fungus.

tinea pedis: Also known as athlete's foot; an infection of the foot caused by a fungus.

Tinel's sign: A special test for the presence of nerve injury or dysfunction in which the examiner "taps" over a superficial nerve such as the ulnar nerve in the ulnar groove, the median nerve in the carpal tunnel, the common peroneal as it wraps around the head of the fibula of the tibial nerve as it crosses posterior to the medial malleolus. A normal "twinge" or brief tingling sensation is a negative test.

tinnitus: Ringing in the ears.

tissue hypoxia: Lack of oxygen to the tissues.

toe-off: The point following midstance when the weight is transferred to the toes and just before the foot leaves the ground.

tone: The normal tension of a relaxed muscle.

tonic (clonic): An unremitting muscular contraction.

tonsillectomy: The surgical removal of the tonsils.

tonsillitis: Inflammation of the tonsils.

tonsils: Any group of lymphoid tissue. Commonly we refer to the tonsils as the lymphoid tissue located bilaterally in the back of the throat.

torque: The product of force times distance. All rotary motions produce torque. In joint motions, torque is the product of muscular force times the perpendicular distance from the line of the force's action to the axis of rotation.

torque arm: *See* force arm.

torsion: Twisting action; tibial torsion is a rotation of the tibia about the longitudinal axis relative to the position of the femur; femoral torsion is a rotation of the femur about the longitudinal axis relative to the position of the tibia.

torticollis: A cervical muscle spasm causing pain, stiffness, and a characteristic lateral flexion of the neck.

tourniquet: A device that encircles a limb that is used to temporarily stop the flow of blood or control bleeding to a distal body segment.

toxemia: The presence of toxic levels of bacteria in the blood.

toxic shock syndrome: An acute and sudden staphylococcus disease associated with the use of tampons, characterized by nausea, vomiting, erythema, and shock; sometimes fatal.

trachea: The hollow organ that connects the larynx to the two bronchi of the lungs.

tracheitis: Inflammation of the trachea.

tracheotomy: An opening created directly into the trachea in which a tube is inserted to facilitate respiration.

traction: The use of longitudinal tension to realign body segments.

transcutaneous: Through the skin.

transcutaneous electrical nerve stimulator (TENS): The use of electrical current to cause excitation of the nerves for the purposes of pain control. *See* gate control theory.

transducer: A device that transforms one type of energy to another, such as an ultrasound device that transforms electrical energy into a mechanical sound wave.

transferrin: An iron-transporting protein.

transient ischemic attack (TIA): A mini stroke, often a precursor to cerebrovascular accident. It is a temporary loss of blood supply to the brain causing temporary facial paralysis, numbness, slurred speech, and vision impairment.

transitory paralysis: Temporary paralysis.

transmissible: Referring to disease that can be passed from one person to another.

transplant: A surgical procedure in which an injured or ill organ is replaced with a healthy one.

transverse plane: Divides the body into upper and lower parts. Motions that take place in this plane include internal/external rotation, horizontal abduction/adduction, and trunk and neck rotation.

Trendelenburg's test: Special test of the hip for gluteus medius weakness. *See* Special Tests—Hip (Appendix 16).

triage: A process of classifying ill or injured individuals according to the severity of their conditions and the likelihood of survival.

triceps surae: The two heads of the gastrocnemius and the soleus.

tricuspid: The valve between the left atrium and ventricle.

trigeminal nerve: Cranial nerve V responsible for motor function involved in chewing and facial sensation. *See* Appendix 7.

trigeminal neuralgia: A condition affecting the fifth cranial nerve in which pain is present in the face and jaw.

trigger finger: In impairment, usually affecting the flexor tendon of the third or fourth finger. There is a thickening or a narrowing of the tendon sheath causing the finger to "stick" in a flexed position when unclenching the fist, until suddenly it gives way as if someone released a trigger.

trigger point: A deep, tender, palpable area of tissue that when pressure is applied to it, causes the pattern of pain (sometimes radiating) to be reproduced.

triglyceride: A type of fat found in the blood related to increased incidence of heart disease, high blood pressure, and diabetes.

trochlear nerve: Cranial nerve IV responsible for eye movement along with the abducens and oculomotor nerves. *See* Appendix 7.

true leg length: Real leg length; a measurement from the medial malleolus to the ASIS.

t-test: A statistical test used to compare two sets of parametric data.

tuberculosis: An infectious bacterial disease of the lungs that is transmitted through the air.

tumor: An abnormal malignant or benign mass.

tunnel vision: A disease that causes loss of peripheral vision, commonly caused by glaucoma.

turf toe: A sprain of the first metatarsophalangeal joint.

two-point discrimination: The ability to discriminate fine cutaneous sensations. The examiner uses a two-point discriminator to determine the distance at which the patient can discriminate one point from two.

tympanic membrane: Eardrum.

type I diabetes: Also known as insulin-dependent diabetes mellitus or juvenile-onset diabetes; this is the more severe form, developing in childhood or adolescence and characterized by an inability to properly secrete insulin, causing hyperglycemia and potentially ketoacidosis.

type II diabetes: Also called adult-onset noninsulin-dependent diabetes mellitus; this is the most common form of diabetes, characterized by hyperglycemia as a result of inadequate production and utilization of insulin.

type I error: The rejection of the null hypothesis when, in fact, the null is true.

type II error: Acceptance of the null hypothesis when, in fact, the null is false.

type I fiber: Slow twitch fiber; slow oxidative fiber; takes twice as long as the fast twitch fibers to reach maximum tension but is more resistant to fatigue.

type II fiber: Fast twitch fiber; fast oxidative fiber; twice as fast as the type I at reaching maximum tension; capable of very quick, forceful contractions but fatigues quicker than type I.

ulcer: An open sore of the skin or mucous membrane, often referring to the lining of the stomach.

ulcerative colitis: Ulcers of the colon and rectum.

ulnar nerve: One of the terminal branches of the brachial plexus arising from the medial cord of the brachial plexus. The ulnar nerve crosses the elbow posterolaterally through the ulnar groove and courses anteromedially along the ulnar side of the anterior forearm and supplies the medial palmar.

ultrasound: A therapeutic modality that uses sound waves.

ultrasound scanning: Sonography; the use of sound waves as a diagnostic process to view the internal organs.

ultraviolet (UV): An electromagnetic radiation that is beyond the visible light with a wavelength in the range of 180 to 390 nanometers. UV is used therapeutically to treat skin conditions.

umbilical hernia: A weak area in the abdominal wall, present at birth, in which the baby's intestines protrude through the wall near the umbilicus.

undescended testicle: A testicle that has not developed into the scrotum and is still located in the abdomen.

unilateral: Relating to only one side of the body.

universal precautions: A procedure for handling bodily fluids recommended by the Centers for Disease Control and Prevention in 1985 and updated in 1996. *See* Appendix 17.

unsaturated fat: A type of fat or oil found mainly in vegetables.

upper motor neuron lesion (UMNL): Injury or illness in the corticospinal or pyramidal tract of the brain or spinal cord resulting in hemi-, para-, or quadriplegia. Symptoms include spasticity, paralysis, positive Babinski, and other pathological reflexes.

urea: Protein waste product that is created in the liver and released by the kidneys.

uremia: An abnormally high level of urea in the blood.

ureters: Bilateral tubes from the kidneys to the bladder.

urethra: The passageway from the bladder in which urine is released.

urethritis: Inflammation of the urethra.

urethrocele: A condition in which the urethra bulges into the vagina.

urethrocystitis: Inflammation of the urethra and the bladder.

urinalysis: The chemical assessment of the urine.

urinary incontinence: The inability to control the release of urine.

urinary tract: Includes the kidneys, ureters, bladder, and urethra.

uterus: The area in which the fetus develops following the fertilization of the egg.

uvea: The middle layer of the eye consisting of colored area just below the sclera.

uveitis: Inflammation of the uvea.

V

vaccination: A form of immunization in which antibodies to a particular disease are developed in the body in response to the introduction of a weakened from of a microorganism. The development of the antibodies will protect the body in the event that there is an exposure to the microorganisms.

vaginitis: Inflammation of the vagina characterized by itching and burning sensations.

vagus nerve: Cranial nerve X responsible for breathing, swallowing, and sensation of the larynx, pharynx, and bronchii. *See* Appendix 7.

valgus: A deformity in which the distal end of a bone deviates laterally, such as "knock knees"; also known as genu (knee) valgum.

valgus stress: The application of ligamentous stress applied to the lateral aspect of the limb forcing the limb into a valgus position.

validity: The soundness of a measurement technique to measure what it was intended to measure.

Valsalva's maneuver: A special test for nerve involvement. *See* Special Tests—Spine (Appendix 16).

variance: The average of the squared deviations from the mean.

varicella: Chickenpox.

varicocele: Varicose veins on the testicles.

varicose veins: Enlarged or inflamed veins near the surface of the skin, often causing discomfort or pain.

variola: Smallpox.

varus: A deformity in which the distal end of a bone deviates medially, such as "bowlegged"; also known as genu (knee) varum.

varus stress: The application of ligamentous stress applied to the medial aspect of the limb forcing the limb into a varus position.

vas deferens: A small passageway that stores and transports sperm.

vascular: Relating to blood vessels.

vasculitis: Inflammation of the blood vessels.

vasectomy: A surgical procedure in which the vas deferens are cut and tied off so that sperm will no longer be present in the semen; sterilization.

vasoconstriction: A process in which there is a narrowing of blood vessels.

vasodilation: A process in which there is an opening or widening of blood vessels.

vasospasm: A constriction of a blood vessel reducing blood flow.

vasovagal attack: A sudden loss of consciousness due to a decrease in heart rate.

vein: A blood vessel responsible for carrying the blood back to the heart.

venereal disease (VD): Any sexually transmitted disease.

ventilator: An apparatus that provides breathing for a person who cannot breathe on his or her own.

ventricle: A chamber responsible for the circulation of fluid; the heart contains a left and right ventricle responsible for pumping blood through the body; the brain contains four ventricles which pump cerebrospinal fluid throughout the brain.

ventricular fibrillation: Irregular contractions of the heart in which the heart is "out of sync" and not effective in circulating blood.

verruca: Wart.

vertebra: A small, irregular-shaped bone of the spine; there are 33 bones that make up the spine: 7 cervical, 12 thoracic, 5 lumbar, 5 sacral, and 4 coccygeal.

vertigo: Dizziness.

very low-density lipoprotein (VLDL): A blood protein that is associated with heart disease.

ler used to treat asthma through its
he bronchioles.
 dry skin.
ohy.

vesicle: A small, fluid-filled sac.

vestibulocochlear nerve: Cranial nerve VIII responsible for hearing and balance. *See* Appendix 7.

viral: Pertaining to a virus.

virus: A disease-causing microorganism that reproduces itself only when it resides inside the cell of another organism.

viscoelastic: A substance possessing both viscous and elastic properties.

viscosity: The thickness of a fluid; the resistance to flow of a fluid.

visual acuity: A measure of the sharpness or clarity of vision.

visual field: Peripheral vision.

vitamin: A natural compound essential to proper nutrition and regulation of metabolism found in natural foodstuffs and produced within the body.

vitreous humor: The clear, watery fluid found behind the lens of the eye.

VLDL: *See* very low-density lipoprotein.

volar: Pertaining to the palm of the hand or sole of the foot.

Volkman's contracture: A contracture of the forearm flexors due to ischemia; a possible complication of forearm fracture.

volume: The space occupied by an object.

vulvovaginitis: Inflammation of the vulva and vagina.

W

wart: Verruca; a rough benign growth of the skin caused by a virus.

Watson test: A special test for lunate/scaphoid subluxation. *See* Special Tests—Hand/Wrist (Appendix 16).

watt: The unit of electrical power; a measure of power equal to the power of one amp traveling across a potential difference of one volt; the unit of measure for ultrasound intensity.

wave: An oscillation with a defined frequency, duration, and amplitude.

waveform: In therapeutic modalities, the shape of the wave; examples include sine, square, triangular, asymmetrical, and twin peak.

wavelength: The distance from the beginning to the end of one complete waveform usually measured from the top of one wave to the same point on the top of the next.

weight: The force of gravity on a mass.

weightbearing exercise: Exercises that are performed under the stress of one's body weight.

well straight-leg raise: Special test of the lumbar spine for nerve root compression. *See* Special Tests—Spine (Appendix 16).

wheezing: A symptom of asthma and other respiratory distress syndromes in which a raspy or high-pitched sound is created due to the narrowing of the air passageway.

whiplash injury: A generic term for a neck sprain/strain that was caused by a sudden, forceful extension, followed by flexion similar to that which would occur in a vehicle accident when hit from behind.

white blood cell (WBC): The blood cells that are responsible for helping to prevent and fight off infection.

William's flexion ex
emphasize flexior
(knee to chest), ar
erbate symptoms

within normal lim
used to describ
muscle test, or o

Wolff''s law: Law tl
the demands pl;
to stress will al
hypertrophy.

work: The force f
applied. w = f

Xanthine
action
xeroderm
x-ray: *See*

yeast infection: Relating to a candidiasis infection.

Yergason's test: A special test of the shoulder to determine the presence of biceps tendonitis or biceps tendon subluxation. *See* Special Tests—Shoulder (Appendix 16).

Yeoman's test: A special test of the lumbar spine, hip, and/or sacroiliac joint. *See* Special Tests—SI Joint (Appendix 16).

yield point: Elastic limit; the point on a stress-strain curve at which further stress will cause permanent deformation.

BIBLIOGRAPHY

Bantam Medical Dictionary. New York, NY: Bantam Books Inc; 1982.

Bottomley JM. *Quick Reference Dictionary for Physical Therapy.* Thorofare, NJ: SLACK Incorporated; 2000.

Cantu RC. Return to play guidelines after head injury. *Clin Sports Med.* 1998;17:45-60.

Colorado Medical Society and Sports Medicine Committee. Guidelines for the management of concussion in sports. *Colo Med.* 1990;87:4.

Guskiewicz, KM, Perrin, DH. Research and clinical applications of assessing balance. *Journal of Sport Rehabilitation.* 1996;5:45-63.

Harmon KG. Assessment and management of concussion in sports. *Am Fam Physician.* 1999;60:887-94.

Houglum PA. *Therapeutic Exercise for Athletic Injuries.* Champaign, Ill: Human Kinetics; 2001.

Jacobs K, Jacobs L. *Quick Reference Dictionary for Occupational Therapy.* 3rd ed. Thorofare, NJ: SLACK Incorporated; 2001.

King MA. Core stability: Creating a foundation for functional rehabilitation. *Athletic Therapy Today.* 2000; 5(2):6-13.

King MA. Functional stability for the upper quarter. *Athletic Therapy Today.* 2000; 5(2):17-21.

Knight KL. Guidelines for rehabilitation of sports injuries. *Clin Sports Med.* 1985; 4:405-416.

Kreighbaum E, Barthels KM. *Biomechanics: A Qualitative Approach for Studying Human Movement.* 3rd ed. New York, NY: Macmillan; 1990.

LeVeau BF. *Biomechanics of Human Motion.* Philadelphia, Pa: WB Saunders; 1992.

Magee DJ. *Orthopedic Physical Assessment.* 3rd ed. Philadelphia, Pa: WB Saunders; 1997.

McCrea M, Kelly JT, Randolph C. *The standardized assessment of concussion (SAC): Manual for administration, scoring, and interpretation.* Washington, DC: Brain Injury Association; 1997.

McGinnis PM. *Biomechanics of Sport and Exercise.* Champaign, Ill: Human Kinetics; 1999.

NATA. *Blood Borne Pathogens Guidelines for Athletic Trainers. Position Statement of the National Athletic Trainers' Association.* Dallas, Tex: NATA; 1995.

NATA. *Code of Ethics.* Dallas, Tex: National Athletic Trainers' Association. Dallas, Tex: NATA; 2000.

NATA. *Membership Policies and Privileges.* Dallas, Tex: National Athletic Trainers' Association. Dallas, Tex: NATA; 2000.

NATABOC. *Credentialing Information.* Dallas, Tex: NATABOC; 2000.

NATABOC. *Standards of Professional Practice.* Dallas, Tex: NATABOC; 2000.

Prentice WE. *Rehabilitation Techniques in Sports Medicine.* 3rd ed. Boston, Mass: McGraw Hill Companies Inc.; 1999.

Prentice WE. *Therapeutic Modalities in Sports Medicine.* 4th ed. Boston, Mass: McGraw Hill Companies Inc.; 1999.

Prentice WE, Arnheim DD. *Principles of Athletic Training.* 10th ed. Boston, Mass: McGraw Hill Companies Inc.; 2000.

Random House Webster's Dictionary. 2nd ed. New York, NY: Random House Incorporated; 1996.

Riemann BL, Guskiewicz KM. Relationship between clinical and forceplate measures of postural stability. *Journal of Sport Rehabilitation.* 1999; 8(2):1-7.

Schultz SJ, Houglum PA, Perrin DH. *Assessment of Athletic Injuries.* Champaign, Ill: Human Kinetics; 2001.

Starkey C. *Therapeutic Modalities for Athletic Trainers.* Philadelphia, Pa: FA Davis; 1993.

Starkey C, Ryan J. *Evaluation of Orthopedic and Athletic Injuries.* Philadelphia, Pa: FA Davis; 1996.

Stedman's Concise Medical Dictionary for the Health Professions. 3rd ed. Baltimore, Md: Williams & Wilkins; 1997.

Taber's Cyclopedic Medical Dictionary. 19th ed. Philadelphia, Pa: FA Davis; 2001.

Vincent WJ. *Statistics in Kinesiology.* Champaign, Ill: Human Kinetics; 1995.

LIST OF APPENDICES

APPENDIX 1

Medical Roots Terminology

Reprinted with permission from Bottomley J. *Quick Reference Dictionary for Physical Therapy*. Thorofare, NJ: SLACK Incorporated; 2000.

a-	negative prefix; eg, ametria (n is added before words beginning with a vowel)
ab-	away from; eg, abducent
abdomin-	abdomen; eg, abdominis, abdominoscopy
ac-	*see* ad-; eg, accretion
ac-	pertaining to
acet-	acid; eg, acetum vinegar, acetometer
acid-	acid; eg, acidus sour, aciduric
acou-	hear; eg, acouesthesia (also spelled acu-)
act-	drive, act; eg, reaction
actin-	ray, radius; eg, actinogenesis
acr-	extremity, peak; eg, acromegaly
acu-	hear; eg, osteoacusis
ad-	toward (d changes to c, f, g, p, s, or t before words beginning with those consonants); eg, adrenal
aden-	gland; eg, adenoma
adeno-	gland
adip-	fat; eg, adipocellular, adipose
-aemia	blood; eg, polycythaemia
aer-	air; eg, anaerobiosis
aero-	air
aesthe-	sensation; eg, aesthesioneurosis
af-	*see* ad-; eg, afferent
ag-	*see* ad-; eg, agglutinant
-agogue	leading, inducing; eg, galactagogue
-agra	catching, seizure; eg, podagra

al-	pertaining to white; eg, albocinereous
albo-	white
alg-	pain; eg, neuralgia, algesia
all-	other, different; eg, allergy
alve-	channel, cavity; eg, alveolar, alveous trough
amb-	both, on both sides; eg, ambulate
amph-	*see* amphi-, around, on both sides; eg, ampheclexis
amphi-	both, doubly (i is dropped before words beginning with a vowel); eg, amphicelous
amyl-	starch; eg, amylosynthesis
an-	pertaining to
an-	*see* ana-; eg, anagogic
ana-	up, positive (final a is dropped before words beginning with a vowel); eg, anaphoresis
andr-	man; eg, gynandroid
angi-	vessel; eg, angiemphraxis
angio-	vessel
ankyl-	crooked, looped; eg, ankylodactylia (also spelled ancyl-)
ant-	*see* anti-, antophthalmic
ante-	before; eg, anteflexion
anti-	against, counter (i is dropped before words beginning with a vowel or the word is hyphenated); eg, antipyogenic, anti-inflammatory (*see also* contra-)
antr-	cavern; eg, antrodynia
ap-	*see* ad-; eg, append
-aph-	touch; eg, dysaphia (*see also* hapt-)
apo-	away from, detached, opposed (o is dropped before words beginning with a vowel); eg, apophysis
ar-	pertaining to
arachn-	spider; eg, arachnodactyly

arch-	beginning, origin; eg, archenteron
arter(i)-	elevator, artery; eg, arteriosclerosis, periarteritis
arthr-	joint; eg, synarthrosis (*see also* articul-)
arthro-	joint
articul-	articulus joint; eg, disarticulation (*see also* arthr-)
as-	*see* ad-; eg, assimilation
-ase	enzyme
at-	*see* ad-; eg, attrition
audio-	hearing
aur-	ear; eg, aurinasal (*see also* ot-)
aut-	self; eg, autechoscope
auto-	self; eg, autoimmune
aux-	increase; eg, enterauxe
ax-	axis; eg, axofugal
axon-	axis; eg, axonometer
ba-	go, walk, stand; eg, hypnobatia
bacill-	small staff, rod; eg, actinobacillosis (*see also* bacter-)
bacter-	small staff, rod; eg, bacteriophage (*see also* bacill-)
ball-	throw; eg, ballistics (*see also* bol-)
bar-	weight; eg, pedobarometer
bi-	life; eg, aerobic
bi-	two, twice, double; eg, bipedal
bil-	bile; eg, biliary
bio-	life
blast-	bud, child, a growing thing in its early stages; eg, blastoma, zygotoblast
blep-	look; eg, hemiablepsia
blephar-	eyelid; eg, blepharoncus
bol-	ball; eg, embolism
brachi-	arm; eg, brachiocephalic
brachy-	short; eg, brachycephalic
brady-	slow; eg, bradycardia

brom-	stench; eg, podobromidrosis
bronch-	windpipe; eg, bronchoscopy
bry-	be full of life; eg, embryonic
bucc-	cheek; eg, distobuccal
cac-	bad, evil, abnormal; eg, cacodontia, arthrocace (*see also* mal-, dys-)
calc-	stone, limestone, lime; eg, calcipexy
calc-	heel; eg, calcaneotibial
calor-	heat; eg, calorimeter (*see also* therm-)
cancr-	cancer, crab; eg, cancrology (*see also* carcin-)
capit-	head; eg, decapitate (*see also* cephal-)
caps-	container; eg, encapsulation
carbo-	coal, charcoal; eg, carbohydrate, carbonuria
carcin-	crab, cancer; eg, carcinoma (*see also* cancr-)
cardi-	heart; eg, lipocardiac
cardio-	heart
cat-	*see* cata-; eg, cathode
cata-	down, negative (final a is dropped before words beginning with a vowel); eg, catabatic
caud-	tail; eg, caudate
cav-	hollow; eg, concave
cec-	blind; eg, cecopexy
-cele	tumor, hernia, cyst; eg, gastrocele
cell-	room; eg, celliferous
cen-	common; eg, cenesthesia
cent-	one hundred; eg, centimeter, centipede
cente-	puncture; eg, enterocentesis, amniocentesis
centr-	central point, center; eg, neurocentral
cephal-	relating to the head; eg, encephalitis
cept-	take, receive; eg, receptor
cer-	wax; eg, ceroplasty, ceromel

cerebr-	relating to the cerebrum; eg, cerebrospinal
cervic-	neck; eg, cervicitis, cervical
chancr-	crab, cancer; eg, chancriform
chir-	hand; eg, chiromegaly
chlor-	green; eg, achloropsia
chloro-	green
chol-	bile; eg, hepatocholangeitis
chondr-	cartilage; eg, chondromalcia
chondro-	cartilage
chord-	string, cord; eg, perichordal
chori-	protective fetal membrane; eg, endochorion
chrom-	color; eg, polychromatic
chron-	time; eg, synchronous
chy-	pour; eg, ecchymosis
-cid(e)	causing death, cut, kill; eg, infanticide, germicidal
cili-	eyelid; eg, superciliary (*see also* blephar-)
cine-	move; eg, autocinesis
-cipient	take, receive; eg, incipient
circum-	around; eg, circumferential (*see also* peri-)
-cis-	cut, kill; eg, excision
clas-	break; eg, osteoclast, cranioclast
clin-	bend, incline, make lie down; eg, clinometer
clus-	shut; eg, maloclusion
co-	*see* con-; eg, cohesion
cocc-	seed, pill; eg, gonococcus
coel-	hollow; eg, coelenteron (also spelled cel-)
col-	before l; com- before b, m, or p; cor- before r); eg, contraction
col-	pertaining to the lower intestine; eg, colic

col-	*see* con-; eg, collapse
colic-	large intestines
colon-	lower intestine; eg, colonic
colp-	hollow, vagina; eg, endocolpitis
com-	*see* con-; eg, commasculation
con-	with, together (becomes co- before vowels or h;
contra-	against, counter; eg, contraindication (*see also* anti-)
copr-	dung; eg, coproma (*see also* sterco-)
cor-	doll, little image, pupil; eg, isocoria
cor-	*see* con-; eg, corrugator
corpor-	body; eg, intracorporal (*see also* somat-)
cortic-	bark, rind; eg, corticosterone
cost-	rib; eg, intercostal (*see also* pleur-)
crani-	skull, cranium; eg, pericranium
cranio-	skull
creat-	meat, flesh; eg, creatorrhea
-crescent	grow; eg, excrescent
cret-	grow; eg, accretion
cret-	distinguish, separate off; eg, discrete
crin-	distinguish, separate off; eg, endocrinology
crur-	shin, leg; eg, brachiocrural
cry-	cold; eg, cryesthesia
crypt-	hide, conceal; eg, cryptorchism
cult-	tend, cultivate; eg, culture
cune-	wedge; eg, sphencuneiform
cut-	skin; eg, subcutaneous (*see also* derm[at]-)
cyan-	blue; eg, anthocyanin
cycl-	circle, cycle; eg, cyclophoria
cyst-	bag, bladder; eg, nephrocystitis (*see also* vesic-)
cyt-	cell; eg, plasmocytoma (*see also* cell-)
cyto	cell

dacry-	tear; eg, dacryocyst
dactyl-	finger, toe, digit; eg, hexadactylism
de-	down from; eg, decomposition
dec-	ten, indicates multiple in metric system; eg, decagram
dec-	ten, indicates fraction in metric system; eg, decimeter
deci-	tenth; eg, decibel
demi-	half; eg, demipenniform
dendr-	tree; eg, neurodendrite
dent-	tooth; eg, interdental (*see also* odont-)
dento-	teeth
derm-	skin; eg, endoderm, dermatitis (*see also* cut-)
derma-	skin
desm-	band, ligament; eg, syndesmopexy
dextr-	handedness; eg, ambidextrous
di-	two; eg, dimorphic (*see also* bi-2)
di-	*see* dia-; eg, diuresis
di-	*see* dis-; eg, divergent
dia-	through, apart, between, asunder (a is dropped before words beginning with a vowel); eg, diagnosis
didym-	twin, gemini; eg, epididymal
digit-	finger, toe; eg, digital (*see also* dactyl-)
diplo-	double; eg, diplomyelia
dips-	thirst
dis-	apart, away from, negative, absence of (s may be dropped before a word beginning with a consonant); eg, dislocation
disc-	disk; eg, discoplacenta
dors-	back; eg, ventrodorsal
drom-	course; eg, hemodromometer
-ducent	lead, conduct; eg, adducent
duct-	lead, conduct; eg, oviduct
dur-	hard, sclera; eg, induration
dynam(i)-	power; eg, dynamoneure, neurodynamic

-dynia	pain; eg, coxodynia
dys-	bad, improper, malfunction, difficult; eg, dystrophic
e-	out from; eg, emission
-eal	pertaining to
ec-	out of, on the outside; eg, eccentric
-ech-	have, hold, be; eg, synechotomy
ect-	outside; eg, ectoplasm (*see also* extra-)
ecto-	out, without, away
-ectomy	a cutting out; eg, mastectomy
ede-	swell; eg, edematous
ef-	out of; eg, efflorescent
-elc-	sore, ulcer; eg, enterelcosis (*see also* helc-)
electr-	amber; eg, electrotherapy
em-	in, on; eg, embolism, empathy, emphlysis (*see also* en-)
-em-	blood; eg, anemia (*see also* hem[at]-)
-emesis	vomiting; eg, nemesis
-emia	blood; eg, bacteremia
en-	in, on, into (n changes to m before b, p, or ph); eg, encelitis
encephal-	brain
end-	inside; eg, endangium (*see also* intra-)
endo-	within; eg, endocardium
enter-	intestine; eg, dysentery
epi-	upon, after, in addition (i is dropped before words beginning with a vowel); eg, epiglottis, epaxial
erg-	work, deed; eg, energy
erythr-	red, rubor; eg, erythrochromia
erythro-	red
eso-	inside; eg, esophylactic (*see also* intra-, endo-)
esthe-	perceive, feel, sensation; eg, anesthesia
eu-	good, normal, well; eg, eupepsia, eugeric

ex-	out of; eg, excretion
exo-	outside; eg, exopathic (*see also* extra-)
extra-	outside of, beyond; eg, extracellular
faci-	face; eg, brachiofaciolingual
-facient	make; eg, calefacient
-fact-	make; eg, artefact
fasci-	band; eg, fascia
febr-	fever; eg, febrile, febricide
-fect-	make; eg, defective
-ferent	bear, carry; eg, efferent, afferent
ferr-	iron; eg, ferroprotein
fibr-	fiber; eg, chondofibroma
fibro-	fiber
fil-	thread; eg, filament, filiform
fiss-	split; eg, fissure
flagell-	whip; eg, flagellation
flav-	yellow; eg, riboflavin
-flect-	bend, divert; eg, deflection
-flex-	bend, divert; eg, reflexometer, flexion
flu-	flow; eg, fluid
flux-	flow; eg, affluxion
for-	door, opening; eg, foramen, perforated
fore-	before, in front of; eg, forefront
-form	shape, form; eg, ossiform, cuniform
fract-	break; eg, fracture, refractive
front-	forehead, front; eg, nasofrontal
-fug(e)	to drive away, flee, avoid; eg, vermifuge, centrifugal
funct-	perform, serve, function; eg, functional, malfunction
fund-	pour; eg, infundibulum
fus-	pour; eg, diffusible
galact-	milk; eg, dysgalactia
gam-	marriage, reproductive union; eg, agamont

gangli-	swelling, plexus; eg, neurogangliitis
gastro-	stomach, belly; eg, gastrostomy
gelat-	freeze, congeal; eg, gelatin
gemin-	twin, double; eg, quadrigeminal
gen-	become, be produced, originate, formation; eg, genesis, cytogenic, gene
-genesis	beginning
germ-	bud, a growing thing in its early stages; eg, germinal, ovigerm
gest-	bear, carry; eg, congestion
gland-	acorn; eg, intraglandular
-glia	glue; eg, neuroglia
gloss-	relating to the tongue; eg, lingutrichoglossia
glott-	tongue, language; eg, glottic
gluc-	sweet; eg, glucose
glutin-	glue; eg, agglutination
glyco-	sugar
glyc(y)-	sweet; eg, glycemia, glycyrrhia
gnath-	jaw; eg, orthognathous
gno-	know, discern; eg, diagnosis
gon-	produce, formulate; eg, gonad, amphigony
grad-	walk, take steps; eg, retrograde
-gram	scratch, write, record; eg, cardiogram
gran-	grain, particle; eg, lipogranuloma, granulation
graph-	scratch, write, record; eg, histography
grav-	heavy; eg, multigravida
gyn(ec)-	woman, wife; eg, androgyny, gynecologic
gyr-	ring, circle; eg, gyrospasm
haem(at)-	pertaining to blood; eg, haemorrhagia, haematoxylon
hapt-	touch; eg, haptometer
hect-	one hundred, indicates multiple in metric system; eg, hectometer

helc-	sore, ulcer; eg, helcosis
hem(at)-	blood; eg, hematocyturia, hemangioma
hemi	half; eg, hemiageusia (*see also* semi-)
hemo-	blood
hen-	one; eg, henogenesis
hepat-	liver; eg, gastrohepatic
hept(a)-	seven; eg, heptatomic, heptavalent
hered-	heir; eg, heredity
hetero-	other, indicating dissimilarity; eg, heterogeneous
hex-	six, sex-, hexly-; eg, hexagram
hex-	have, hold, be; eg, cachexy
hexa-	six, sex-, hexly-; eg, hexachromic
hidr-	sweat; eg, hyperhidrosis
hist-	web, tissue; eg, histodialysis
hod-	road, path; eg, hodoneuromere
holo-	all; eg, hologenesis
homo-	common, same; eg, homomorphic
horm-	impetus, impulse; eg, hormone
hydat-	water; eg, hydatism
hydr-	pertaining to water; eg, achlorhydria
hydro-	water
hyp-	under; eg, hypaxial, hypodermic
hyper-	over, above, beyond, extreme; e.g., hypertrophy
hypn-	sleep; e.g., hypnotic
hypo-	under, below (o is dropped before words beginning with a vowel); eg, hypometabolism
hyster-	womb; eg, hysterectomy
-ia	condition of
-iasis	condition, pathological state; eg, hemiathriasis (*see also* -osis)
iatr-	specialty in medicine; eg, pediatrics
-ic	pertaining to
idio-	peculiar, separate, distinct; eg, idiosyncrasy

il-	negative prefix (eg, illegible); in, on (eg, illinition)
ile-	pertaining to the ileum (ile- is commonly used to refer to the portion of the intestines known as the ileum); eg, ileostomy
ili-	lower abdomen, intestines, (ili- is commonly used to refer to the flaring part of the hip bone known as the ilium); eg, iliosacral
im-	in, on (eg, immersion); negative prefix (eg, imperfection)
in-	fiber; eg, inosteatoma
in-	in, on (n changes to l, m, or r before words beginning with those consonants); eg, insertion
in-	negative prefix; eg, invalid
infra-	beneath; eg, infraorbital
insul-	island; eg, insulin
inter-	among, between; eg, intercarpal
intra-	inside; eg, intravenous
ir-	in, on (eg, irradiation); negative prefix (eg, irreducible)
irid-	rainbow, colored circle; eg, keratoiridocyclitis
is-	equal; eg, isotope
ischi-	hip, haunch; eg, ischiopubic
-ism	condition, theory; eg, hemiballism, agism
iso-	equal; eg, isotonic
-ist	specialist
-itis	inflammation; eg, neuritis
-ive	pertaining to
-ize	to treat by special method; eg, specialize
jact-	throw; eg, jactitation

ject-	throw; eg, injection
jejun-	hungry, not partaking of food; eg, gastrojejunostomy
jug-	yoke; eg, conjugation
junct-	yoke, join; eg, conjunctiva
juxta-	near; eg, juxtaposed
kary-	nut, kernel, nucleus; eg, megakaryocyte
kerat-	horn; eg, keratolysis, keratin
kil-	one thousand, indicates multiple in metric system; eg, kilogram
kine-	move; eg, kinematics
kinesio-	movement
-kinesis	movement; eg, orthokinesis
labi-	lip; eg, gingivolabial
lact-	milk; eg, glucolactone, lactose
lal-	talk, babble; eg, glossolalia
lapar-	flank, loin, abdomen; eg, laparotomy
laryng-	windpipe; eg, laryngendoscope
lat-	ear, carry; eg, translation
later-	side; eg, bentrolateral
lent-	lentil; eg, lenticonus
lep-	take, seize; eg, cataleptic, epileptic
lepto-	small, soft; eg, leptotene
leuk-	white; eg, leukocyte (also spelled leuc-)
lien-	spleen; eg, lienocele
lig-	tie, bind; eg, ligate
lingu-	tongue; eg, sublingual
lip-	fat; eg, glycolipid
lipo-	fat
lith-	stone; eg, nephrolithotomy
litho-	stone
loc-	place; eg, locomotion
log-	speak, give an account; eg, logorrhea, embryology

-logy	study of
lumb-	loin; eg, dorsolumbar
lute-	yellow; eg, xanthluteoma
ly-	loose, dissolve; eg, keratolysis
-lysis	setting free, disintegration; eg, glycolysis
lymph-	water; eg, hydrolymphadenosis
macro-	long, large; eg, marcromyoblast
mal-	bad, abnormal; eg, malfunction
malac-	soft; eg, osteomalacia
mamm-	breast; eg, mammogram, mammary
man-	hand; eg, maniphalanx, manipulation
mani-	mental aberration; eg, kleptomania
-mania	excessive preoccupation
mast-	breast; eg, mastectomy, hypermastia
medi-	middle; eg, medial, medifrontal
mega-	great, large, indicates multiple (1 million) in metric system; eg, megacolon, megadyne
megal-	great, large; eg, cardiomegaly, acromegaly
mel-	limb, member; eg, symmelia
melan-	black; eg, melanoma, melanin
melano-	black
men-	month; eg, menopause, dysmenorrhea
mening-	membrane; eg, encephalomeningitis
ment-	mind; eg, dementia
mer-	part; eg, polymeric
mes-	middle; eg, mesoderm
meso-	middle
met-	after, beyond, accompanying; eg, met-allergy
meta-	after, beyond, accompanying (a is dropped before words beginning with a vowel); eg, metacarpal, metatarsal
-meter	measure

metr-	measure; eg, stereometry
metr-	womb; eg, endometritis
micr-	small; eg, photomicrograph
micro-	small
mill-	one thousand, indicates fraction in metric system; eg, milligram, millipede
mio-	smaller, less; eg, mionectic
miss-	send; eg, intromission
-mittent	send; eg, intermittent
mne-	remember; eg, pseudomnesia
mon-	only, sole, single; eg, monoplegia
mono-	single
morph-	form, shape; eg, morphonuclear
mot-	move; eg, vasomotor, locomotion
multi-	many; eg, multiple
my-	muscle; eg, myopathy
-myces	fungus; eg, myelomyces
myc(et)-	fungus; eg, ascomycetes, streptomycin
myel-	marrow; eg, poliomyelitis
myo-	muscle
myx-	mucus; eg, myxedema
narc-	numbness; eg, toponarcosis, narcolepsy
nas-	nose; eg, nasal
necr-	corpse, dead; eg, necrocytosis, necrosis
necro-	dead
neo-	new, young; eg, neocyte, neonate
nephr-	kidney; eg, nephron, nephric
nephro-	kidney
neur-	nerve; eg, neurology, estesioneure
neuro-	nerve and brain
nod-	knot; eg, nodosity
nom-	deal out, distribute, law, custom; eg, nominal, taxonomy
non-	nine, no; eg, nonacosane

nos-	disease; eg, nosology
nucle-	nut, kernel; eg, nucleus, nucleide
nutri-	nourish; eg, malnutrition
ob-	against, toward (b changes to c before words beginning with that consonant) eg, obtuse
oc-	*see* ob-, occlude
ocul-	eye; eg, oculomotor
-od-	road, path; eg, periodic
-ode	road, path; eg, cathode
-ode	form; eg, nematode
odont-	tooth; eg, orthodontia
-odyn-	pain, distress; eg, gastrodynia
-oid	form; eg, hyoid; resembling
-ol	oil; eg, cholesterol
-old	form, shape, resemblance; eg, scaffold
ole-	oil; eg, oleorsin
olig-	few, small; eg, oligospermia
-oma	tumor; eg, blastoma
omo-	shoulder; eg, omosternum
omphal-	navel; eg, periomphalic
onc-	bulk, mass; eg, oncology, hematoncometry
onych-	claw, nail; eg, anonychia
oo-	egg, ovum; eg, perioothecitis
oophor-	pertaining to the ovary; eg, oophorectomy
ophthalm-	eye; eg, ophthalmic
or-	mouth; eg, intraoral
orb-	circle; eg, suborbital
orchi-	testicle; eg, orchiopathy
organ-	implement, instrument; eg, organoleptic
-orrhage	excessive bleeding
-orrhagia	hemorrhage
-orrhaphy	suture

-orrhea	flow, discharge
-orrhexis	rupture
orth-	straight, right, normal; eg, orthopedics
-osis	condition, disease; eg, osteoporosis
oss-	bone; eg, osseous, ossiphone
ost(e)-	bone; eg, enostosis, osteonecrosis
-ostomy	new opening
ot-	ear; eg, parotid (*see also* aur-)
oto-	ear
-otomy	cutting; eg, osteotomy
-ous	pertaining to
ov-	egg; eg, synovia
oxy-	sharp, acid; eg, oxycephalic
pachy(n)-	thicken; eg, pachyderma, myopachynsis
pag-	fix, make fast; eg, thoracopagus
pan-	entire, all; eg, pancytosis, pandemic
par-	bear, give birth to; eg, primiparous
par-	*see* para-; eg, parepigastric
para-	beside, beyond, along side of (final a is dropped before words beginning with a vowel); eg, paramastoid
part-	bear, give birth to; eg, parturition
path-	that which one undergoes, sickness, disease; eg, pathology, psychopathic
patho-	disease
pec-	fix, make fast; eg, sympectothiene (*see also* pex-)
ped-	child; eg, pediatric, orthopedic
pell-	skin, hide; eg, pellagra
-pellent	drive; eg, repellent
pen-	need, lack; eg, erythrocytopenia
pend-	hang down; eg, appendix
-penia	deficiency
pent(a)-	five; eg, pentose, pentaploid
peps-	digest; eg, bradypepsia
pept-	digest; eg, dyspeptic

per-	through, excessive; eg, pernasal
peri-	around; eg, periphery
pet-	seek, tend toward; eg, centripetal
pex-	fix, make fast; eg, hepatopexy
-pexy	fixation
pha-	say, speak; eg, dysphasia
phac-	lentil, lens; eg, phacosclerosis (also spelled phak-)
phag-	eat; eg, lipphagic
phak-	lentil, lens; eg, phakitis
phan-	show, be seen; eg, diaphanoscopy
pharmac-	drug; eg, pharmacology
pharyng-	throat; eg, glossopharyngeal
phen-	show, be seen; eg, phosphene
pher-	bear, support; eg, periphery
phil-	like, have affinity for; eg, eosinophilia, philosophy
phleb-	vein; eg, periphlebitis, phlebotomy
phleg-	burn, inflame; eg, adenophlegmon
-phobia	fear
phlog-	burn, inflame; eg, antiphlogistic
phob-	fear, dread; eg, claustrophobia
phon-	sound; eg, echophony
phono-	voice
phor-	bear, support; eg, exophoria
phos-	light; eg, phosphorus
phot-	light; eg, photerythrous
phrag-	fence, wall off, stop up; eg, diaphragm
phrax-	fence, wall off, stop up; eg, emphraxis
phren-	mind, midriff; eg, metaphrenia, metaphrenon
phthi-	decay, waste away; eg, opthalmophthisis
phy-	beget, bring forth, produce, be by nature; eg, nosophyte, physical
phyl-	tribe, kind; eg, phylogeny
phylac-	guard; eg, prophylactic

-phylaxis	protection; eg, prophylaxis
-phyll	leaf; eg, xanthophyll
phys(a)-	blow, inflate; eg, physocele, physalis
physe-	blow, inflate; eg, emphysema
pil-	hair; eg, epilation
pituit-	phlegm; eg, pituitous
placent-	cake; eg, extraplacental
plas-	mold, shape; eg, cineplasty, plastazode
-plasty	surgical repair
platy-	broad, flat; eg, platyrrhine
pleg-	strike; eg, diplegia, paraplegia
plet-	fill; eg, depletion
pleur-	rib, side; eg, peripleural
plex-	strike; eg, apoplexy
plic-	fold; eg, complication
plur-	more; eg, plural
pne-	breathing; eg, traumatopnea
-pnea	breathing
pneum(at)-	breath, air; eg, pneumodynamics, pneumothorax
pneumo(n)-	lung; eg, pneumocentesis, pneumontomy
pod-	foot; eg, podiatry
poie-	make, produce; eg, sarcopoietic
pol-	axis of a sphere; eg, peripolar
poly-	much, many; eg, polyspermia
pont-	bridge; eg, pontocerebellar
por-	passage; eg, myelopore
por-	callus; eg, porocele
posit-	put, place; eg, deposit, repositor
post-	after, behind in time or place; eg, postnatal, postural
pre-	before in time or place; eg, prenatal, prevesical
press-	press; eg, pressure, pressoreceptive
pro-	before in time or place; eg, progamous, prolapse
proct-	anus; eg, ecteroproctia

prosop-	face; eg, prosopus
proto-	first; eg, prototype
pseud-	false; eg, pseudoparaplegia
psych-	soul, mind; eg, psychosomatic
pto-	fall; eg, nephroptosis
-ptosis	prolapse
pub-	adult; eg, puberty, ischiopubic
puber-	adult; eg, puberty
pulmo(n)-	lung; eg, cardiopulmonary, pulmolith
puls-	drive; eg, propulsion
punct-	prick, pierce; eg, puncture, punctiform
pur-	pus; eg, puration
py-	pus; eg, nephropyosis
pyel-	trough, basin, pelvis; eg, nephropy elitis
pyl-	door, orifice; eg, pylephlebitis
pyo-	pus
pyr-	fire; eg, galactopyra
quadr-	four; eg, quadraplegic, quadrigeminal
quinque-	five; eg, quinquecuspid
rachi-	spine; eg, alorachidian
radi-	ray; eg, irradiation
re-	back, again; eg, retraction
ren-	kidneys; eg, adrenal
ret-	net; eg, retothelium
retro-	backward; eg, retrodeviation, retrograde
rhag-	break, burst; eg, hemorrhagic
rhaph-	suture, stitching; eg, gastrorrhaphy
rhe-	flow, discharge; eg, disrrheal
rhex-	break, burst; eg, metrorrhexis
rhin-	nose; eg, basirhinal
rhino-	nose
rot-	wheel; eg, rotator
rub(r)-	red; eg, bilirubin, rubrospinal

racchar-	sugar; eg, saccharin
sacro-	pertaining to the sacrum; eg, sacroiliac
salping-	tube, trumpet; eg, salpingitis
sanguin-	blood; eg, sanguineous
sarc-	flesh; eg, sarcoma
schis-	split; eg, schistorachis, rachischisis
scler-	hard; eg, sclerosis, scleraderma
sclero-	hardening
scop-	look at, observe; eg, endoscope
sect-	cut; eg, sectile, resection
semi-	half; eg, semiflexion
sens-	perceive, feel; eg, sensory
sep-	rot, decay; eg, sepsis
sept-	fence, wall off, stop up; eg, septal
sept-	seven; eg, septan
ser-	whey, watery substance; eg, serum, serosynovitis
sex-	six; eg, sexdigitate
sial-	saliva; eg, polysialia
sin-	hollow, fold; eg, sinobronchitis
sit-	food; eg, parasitic
solut-	loosen, dissolve, set free; eg, dissolution
-solvent	loosen, dissolve; eg, dissolvent
somat-	body; eg, somatic, psychosomatic
-some	body; eg, dictyosome
spas-	draw, pull; eg, spasm, spastic
spectr-	appearance, what is seen; eg, spectrum, microspectroscope
sperm(at)-	seed; eg, spermacrasia, spermatozoon
spers-	scatter; eg, dispersion
sphen-	wedge; eg, sphenoid
spher-	ball; eg, hemisphere
sphygm-	pulsation; eg, sphygmomanometer
spin-	spine; eg, cerebrospinal
spirat-	breathe; eg, inspiratory
splanchn-	entrails, vicera; eg, neurosplanchnic
splen-	spleen; eg, splenomegaly

spor-	seed; eg, sporophyte, sygospore
squam-	scale; eg, squamus, desquamation
sta-	make stand, stop; eg, genesistasis
stal-	send; eg, peristalsis (*see also* stol-)
staphyl-	bunch of grapes, uvula; eg, staphylococcus, staphylectomy
-stasis	stopping, controlling
stear-	fat; eg, stearodermia
steat-	fat; eg, steatopygous
sten-	narrow, compressed; eg, stenocardia
ster-	solid; eg, cholesterol
sterc-	dung; eg, stercoporphyrin
sthen-	strength; eg, asthenia
stol-	send; eg, diastole
stom(at)-	mouth, orifice; eg, anastomosis, stomatogastric
strep(h)-	twist; eg, strephosymbolia, streptomycin (*see also* stroph-)
strict-	draw tight, compress, cause pain; eg, constriction
-stringent	draw tight, compress, cause pain; eg, astringent
stroph-	twist; eg, astrophic (*see also* strep[h]-)
struct-	pile up (against); eg, obstruction
sub-	under, below (b changes to f or p before words beginning with those consonants); eg, sublumbar
suf-	*see* sub-; eg, suffusion
sup-	*see* sub-; eg, suppository
super-	above, beyond, extreme; eg, supermobility
supra-	above, beyond
sy-	*see* syn-; eg, systole
syl-	*see* syn-; eg, syllepsiology
sym-	*see* syn-; eg, symbiosis, symmetry, sympathetic, symphysis
syn-	with, together (n dropped before s; changes to l before l; and changes to m

before b, m, p, and ph), eg, myosynize
sis

ta-	stretch, put under pressure; eg, ectasis
tac-	order, arrange; eg, atactic
tachy-	over
tact-	touch; eg, contact
tax-	order, arrange; eg, ataxia, taxotomy
tect-	cover; eg, protective
teg-	cover; eg, integument
tel-	end; eg, telosynapsis
tele-	at a distance; eg, teleceptor, telescope
tempor-	time, timely or fatal spot, temple; eg, temporomalar
ten(ont)-	tight stretched band; eg, tenodynia, tenonitis, tenontagra
tens-	stretch; eg, extensor
test-	pertaining to the testicle; eg, testitis
tetra-	four; eg, tetragenous
the-	put, place; eg, synthesis
thec-	repository, case; eg, thecostegnosis
thel-	teat, nipple; eg, thelerethism
thera-	therapy
therap-	treatment; eg, hydrotherapy
therm-	heat; eg, diathermy
thermo-	heat
thi-	sulfur; eg, thiogenic
thorac-	chest; eg, thoracoplasty
thromb-	lump, clot; eg, thrombophlebitits, thrombopenia
thym-	spirit; eg, dysthymia
thyr-	shield, shaped like a door; eg, thyroid
tme-	cut; eg, axonotmesis
toc-	childbirth; eg, dystocia
tom-	cut; eg, appendenctomy
ton-	stretch, put under pressure; eg, tonus, peritoneum
top-	place; eg, topesthesia

tors-	twist; eg, extorsion
tox-	arrow poison, poison; eg, toxemia
trache-	windpipe; eg, tracheotomy
trachel-	neck; eg, tracheloplexy
tract-	draw, drag; eg, protraction
trans-	across; eg, transport
traumat-	wound; eg, traumatic
tri-	three; eg, trigonad
trich-	hair; eg, trichoid
trip-	rub; eg, entripsis
trop-	turn, react; eg, sitotropism
troph-	nurture, relating to nourishment; eg, atrophy
-trophy	nutrition, growth
tuber-	swelling, node; eg, tubercle, tuberculosis
typ-	type; eg, atypical
typh-	for, stupor; eg, adenotyphus
typhl-	blind; eg, typhlectasis
uni-	one; eg, unioval
ur-	urine; eg, polyuria
uro-	urine
vacc-	cow; eg, vaccine
vagin-	sheath; eg, invaginated
vas-	vessel; eg, vascular
ventro-	abdomen, in front of; eg, ventrolateral, ventrose
vers-	turn; eg, inversion
vert-	turn; eg, diverticulum
vesic-	bladder; eg, vesicovaginal
vit-	life; eg, devitalize
vuls-	pull, twitch; eg, convulsion
xanth-	yellow, blond; eg, xanthophyll
xantho-	yellow
-yl-	substance; eg, cacodyl

zo-	life, animal; eg, microzoaria
zyg-	yoke, union; eg, zygote, zygodactyly
zym-	ferment; eg, enzyme

Appendix 2

Acronyms and Abbreviations

(A): assisted
A: assessment, anterior, accommodation
A, Ath: athlete
AAROM: active assistive range of motion
ABD: abduction
AC: acromioclavicular
ac: before meals
ACE: angiotensin converting enzyme
ACL: anterior cruciate ligament
ADA: American Dental Association, American Diabetes Association, American Disabilities Act
ADD: adduction or attention deficit disorder
ADL: activities of daily living
ad lib: as desired
adm: admission
AE: above elbow
AED: automatic external defibrillator
AFO: ankle foot orthosis
AIDS: acquired immunodeficiency syndrome
AIIS: anterior inferior iliac spine
AK: above the knee
ALS: amyotrophic lateral sclerosis
am: morning
AMA: against medical advice
AMA: American Medical Association
Ant: anterior
AP: anterior-posterior
AROM: active range of motion
ART: active resistive training
ASA: aspirin

ASAP: as soon as possible
ASHD: arterial sclerotic heart disease
ASIS: anterior superior iliac spine
assist: assistance
ATC: certified athletic trainer

B: both
(B): bilateral
BE: below elbow
BK: below the knee
BID: twice daily
bilat: bilateral
bm: body mechanics
BM: bowel movement
BMI: body mass index
BPM: beats per minute
BP: blood pressure
BS: blood sugar

C: centrigrade
Ca: carcinoma cancer
CABG: coronary artery bypass graft
CAD: coronary artery disease
Cal: calories
caps: capsules
CBC: complete blood count
CBR: complete bedrest
CC, C/C: chief complaint
cc: cubic centimeter
CD: cardiovascular disease
CDC: Centers for Disease Control and Prevention
CEU: continuing education units
CHF: congestive heart failure
CHI: closed head injury
CIE: clinical instructor educator
cm: centimeter
CNS: central nervous system

c/o: complained of, complains of
COG: center of gravity
COLD: chronic obstructive lung disease
cont: continue
CO$_2$: carbon dioxide
COP: center of pressure
COPD: chronic obstructive pulmonary disease
CP: cerebral palsy, chest pain, cold pack
CPM: continuous passive motion
CPR: cardiopulmonary resuscitation
CPU: central processing unit, computer processing unit
C & S: culture and sensitivity
CSF: cerebrospinal fluid
CV: cardiovascular
CVA: cerebrovascular accident
CWI: crutch walking instructions
CWP: cold whirl pool
Cysto: cystoscopic examination

da or DAW: dispense as written
d/c: discontinued or discharged
Dep: dependent
Dept: department
Derm: dermatology
DHHS: Department of Health and Human Services
DIP: distal interphalangeal joint
DJP: degenerative joint pain
DM: diabetes mellitus
DNR: do not resuscitate
DO: doctor of osteopathy
DOB: date of birth
DTR: deep tendon reflex
DVT: deep vein thrombosis
Dx: diagnosis

EAP: emergency action plan
ECF: extended care facility
ECG, EKG: electrocardiogram

EEG: electroencephalogram
EENT: ear, eye, nose, throat
EIA: exercise-induced asthma
EMG: electromyelogram
EMS: emergency medical services
ENT: ear, nose, throat
ER, E.R.: emergency room
EVAL: evaluation
EX: exercise
EXT: extension

F-: fair (muscle strength, balance)
F/b: followed by
FBS: fasting blood sugar
FH: family history
FLEX: flexion
ft: foot, feet (the measurement, not the body part)
FUO: fever, unknown origin
FWB: full weightbearing
FX: fracture
FY: fiscal year

G: good (muscle strength, balance)
g or gm: gram
GB: gallbladder
GI: gastrointestinal
GTO: golgi tendon organ
GYN: gynecology

H & H, H/H: hematocrit and hemoglobin
H & P: history and physical
HA, H/A: headache
Hb, Hgb: hemoglobin
HBV: hepatitis B virus
Hct: height
HCVD: hypertensive cardiovascular disease
HEENT: head, ear, eye, nose, throat

HI: head injury
HNP: herniated nucleus pulposus
HOB: head of bed
HP: hot pack
HR: heart rate
Hr: hour
hs: at bedtime
Htn: hypertension
Ht: hematocrit
Hx, hx: history
Hz: hertz

IB: ice bag
ICU: intensive care unit
Ila: inferiolateral angle (of the sacrum)
IM: intramuscular
IMP: impression
in: inches
Indep: independent
Inj: injury
I & O: intake and output
IP: interphalangeal
IV: intravenous

JAT: *Journal of Athletic Training*
J Orthop Sports Phys Ther: *Journal of Orthopedic and Sports Physical Therapy*
JSR: *Journal of Sport Rehabilitation*

kcal: kilocalories
kg: kilogram
KJ: knee jerk
KUB: kidney, ureter, bladder

L: liter
(L): left
Lat: lateral
lb: pound

LBP: low back pain
LE: lower extremity
LLE: left lower extremity
LLQ: left lower quadrant
LMN: lower motor neuron
LOC: loss of consciousness
LP: lumbar puncture
LRP: long-range plan
LUE: left upper extremity

M: male
m: meter
ma: milliamperes
Max: maximum
MBD: minimal brain damage
MBI: mild brain injury
MC: metacarpal
MCP: metacarpophalangeal
MD: medical doctor; doctor of medicine
MED: minimum effective dose
Meds: medications
MFT: muscle function test
MFR: myofacial release
mg: milligram
MHI: mild head injury
MI: myocardial infarction
min: minutes
mL: milliliter
mm: millimeter
MMT: manual muscle test
mo: month
Mod: moderate
MRI: magnetic resonance imaging
MS: multiple sclerosis
MTP: metatarsophalangeal

N: normal (muscle strength)
NDT: neurodevelopmental treatment

Neg: negative
N.H.: nursing home
NMES: neuromuscular electrical stimulator
NIH: National Institutes of Health
NMES: neuromuscular electrical stimulator
noc: night, at night
NOCSAE: National Operating Committee on Standards for Athletic Equipment
NPO: nothing by mouth
NSAID: nonsteroidal anti-inflammatory drugs
NSR: normal sinus rhythm
NWB: nonweightbearing

O: objective
OA: osteoarthritis
OBS: organic brain syndrome, observation
OD: once daily
OP: outpatient
OR: operating room
ORIF: open reduction, internal fixation
OT: occupational therapist, occupational therapy
OTC: over the counter
oz: ounce

(p): pain
P: plan (treatment plan), poor (muscle strength, balance)
P.A.: physician's assistant
PA: posterior/anterior
PARA: paraplegia
p.c., pc: after meals
PE: physical examination
PEARLS: pupils, equal and reactive to light simultaneously
per: by or through
per os, PO: by mouth
PERRLA: pupils equal, round, reactive to light and accomodations

PH: past history
PID: pelvic inflammatory disease
PIIS: posterior inferior illiac spine
PIP: proximal interphalangeal joint
PMH: previous medical history
PNF: proprioceptive neuromuscular facilitation
PNI: peripheral nerve injury
POMR: problem-oriented medical record
pos: positive
poss: possible
post: after or behind
Postop: after surgery (operation)
PRE: progressive resistive exercise
Preop: before surgery (operation)
PROM: passive range of motion
prn: whenever necessary
PSIS: posterior superior iliac spine
PT: physical therapy, physical therapist
PT, pt: patient
PTA: physical therapist assistant, prior to admission
PTB: patella tendon bearing
PVD: peripheral vascular disease
PWB: partial weightbearing

q: every
qd: once a day
qh: every hour
qid: four times a day
qn: every night
q2h: every 2 hours
q3h: every 3 hours
q4h: every 4 hours
quart: qt.

(R): right
RA: rheumatoid arthritis
RBC: red blood count

R.D.: registered dietician
re: regarding
Rehab: rehabilitation
resp: respiratory, respiration
RICE: rest, ice, compression, elevation
RICER: rest, ice, compression, elevation, rehabilitation
RLE: right lower extremity
RM: repetition maximum
RN: registered nurse
RO: rule out
ROM: range of motion
ROS: review of systems
RPE: rating of preceived exertion
RROM: resistive range of motion
R.T.: respiratory therapist
RUE: right upper extremity
Rx: treatment prescription, therapy

S & S: signs and symptoms
s/p: status post
SACH: solid ankle cushion heel
SAT: student athletic trainer
SATA: Student Athletic Trainers Association
SCFE: slipped capital femoral epiphysis
SC joint: sternoclavicular joint
sec: seconds
SED: suberythemal dose
SIDS: sudden infant death syndrome
Sig: directions for use, give as follows, let it be labeled
SI(J): sacroiliac (joint)
SLE: systemic lupus erythematosus
SLR: straight leg raise
SNF: skilled nursing facility
SOAP: subjective, objective, assessment, plan
spec: specimen
ST: soft tissue
Stat: immediately, at once

STD: sexually transmitted disease
STM: short-term memory
Sx: symptoms

T: trace (muscle strength)
tab: tablet
TB: tuberculosis
TBI: traumatic brain injury
tbsp, T.: tablespoon
TENS: transcutaneous electrical nerve stimulation
THR: total hip replacement
TIA: transient ischemic attack
TID: three times daily
TKR: total knee replacement
TM(J): temporomandibular (joint)
TNR: tonic neck reflex (also ATNR, STNR)
t.o.: telephone order
TOS: thoracic outlet syndrome
tsp, t.: teaspoon
TTP: tender to palpation
TUR: transurethral resection
Tx: treatment

µa: microamperes
UA: urine analysis
UE: upper extremity
UMN: upper motor neuron
Un: unable
URI: upper respiratory infection
US: ultrasound
ut dict.: as directed
UTI: urinary tract infection
URI: upper respiratory infection

VD: venereal disease
VO: verbal orders (eg, v.o. Dr. Smith/your signature)
Vol: volume
VS: vital signs

WBC: white blood cell count
w/c: wheelchair
W/cm^2: watts per square centimeter
Wk: week
WNL: within normal limits
wt.: weight
WWP: warm whirlpool

x: number of times performed

yd.: yard
y/o: years old
yr.: year

Appendix 3

Symbols

Reprinted with permission from Jacobs K. *Quick Reference Dictionary for Occupational Therapy*. 2nd ed. Thorofare, NJ: SLACK Incorporated; 1999.

↑	increase
↓	decrease
→	to follow
↔	to and from
1°	primary/first degree
2°	secondary/due to/second degree
3°	tertiary/third degree
@	at
α	alpha
β	beta
Δ	delta, change
n	total sample size
N	total population size
μ	micron (former term for micrometer)
π	pi, 3.1416, ratio of circumference of a circle to its diameter
√	root, square root, radical
+	plus, excess, positive
−	minus, deficiency, negative
±	plus or minus, indefinite
~	approximately
≈	approximately equal
=	equals
>	greater than
<	less than
≥	greater than or equal to
≤	less than or equal to
Σ	sum
:	ratio, "is to"
::	equality between ratios, "as"
∴	therefore

$\overline{c}$	with
$\overline{s}$	without
#	number, pound
/	per
♂	male
♀	female

APPENDIX 4

Anatomical Terms of Orientation

anterior: front, ventral

anteroposterior: front to back

caudal: toward the tail (or feet)

cephalad: toward the head

cranial: relating to the head

deep: underneath, further from the surface

distal: further from the beginning, further from the trunk

dorsal: back, posterior

horizontal: parallel to the floor, perpendicular to a vertical line

inferior: below, lower than

lateral: toward the side of the body

medial: toward the midline of the body

posterior: back, dorsal

posteroanterior: from back to front

pronation: internal rotation of the forearm so as to place the palm down

prone: with the front or ventral surface down, lying face down

proximal: closer toward the beginning, closer to the trunk

sagittal: A vertical plane passing through the body from front to back. The midsagittal plane divides the body into left and right halves

superficial: on top, near the surface, shallow

superior: above

supination: external rotation of the forearm so as to place the palm up

supine: with the back or dorsal surface downward, lying face up

transverse: A horizontal plane (parallel to the ground) passing through the body

Ventral: front, anterior

Vertical: upright, perpendicular to horizontal

APPENDIX 5

Muscles of the Body

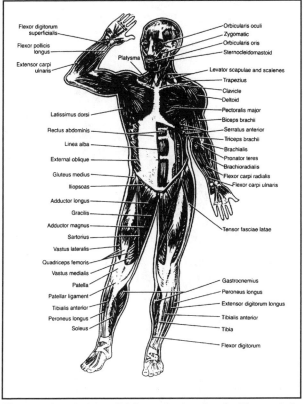

Figure 1. Anterior superficial muscles (reprinted with permission from Leonard P. *Quick and Easy Terminology*. 2nd ed. Philadelphia, Pa: WB Saunders; 1995).

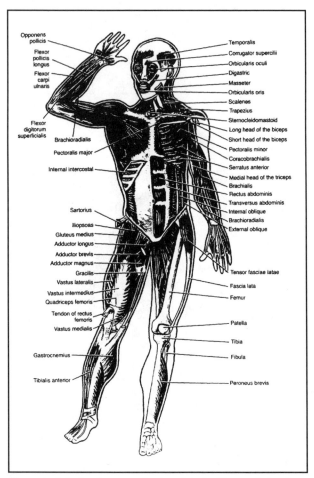

Figure 2. Anterior deep muscles (reprinted with permission from Leonard P. *Quick and Easy Terminology.* 2nd ed. Philadelphia, Pa: WB Saunders; 1995).

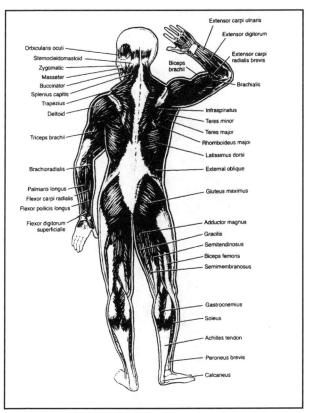

Figure 3. Posterior superficial muscles (reprinted with permission from Leonard P. *Quick and Easy Terminology*. 2nd ed. Philadelphia, Pa: WB Saunders; 1995).

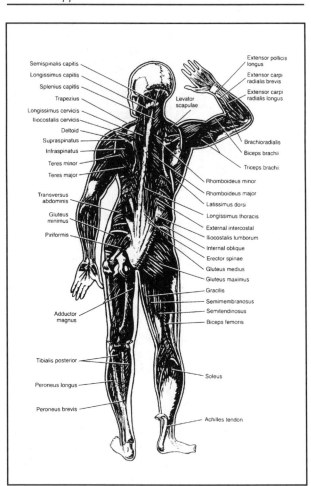

Figure 4. Posterior deep muscles (reprinted with permission from Leonard, P. *Quick and Easy Terminology.* 2nd ed. Philadelphia, Pa: WB Saunders; 1995).

MUSCLES: ORIGIN/INSERTION/ACTION—INNERVATION—BLOOD SUPPLY*

Muscle	Origin	Insertion	Action	Nerve	Artery
Neck					
Sternocleido-mastoid (SCM)	Med or sternal head cranial part of ventral surface of manubrium; lat or clavicular head—sup border & ant surface of med 1/3 clavicle	Lat surface mastoid process & lat 1/2 sup nuchal line of occipital bone	↻ opp side lat ✓ same side ✓ ✓ forward	Spinal accessory n. C2 & C3 ant rami	Subclavian a.
Platysma	Fascia covering sup part of pectoralis major & deltoid	Some fibers into bone below oblique line, others into skin	Draws lip inf & post	Cervical branch of facial n.	Subclavian a. (branch)
Suprahyoid group					
Digastricus	Post belly: mastoid notch of temporal bone; Ant belly: a depression on inner side of inf border of mandible	Post belly: hyoid bone by fibrous loop; Ant belly: same as post belly	▲ hyoid bone Post: draws backwards Ant: draws forward	Post: facial n. Ant: mylohyoid n.	Lingual a.
Stylohyoideus	Post & lat surface of styloid process	Body of hyoid bone	Draws hyoid sup & post	Facial n. (branch)	Lingual a.

*Note: Please refer to key on page 225.

Muscle	Origin	Insertion	Action	Nerve	Artery
Neck					
Mylohyoideus	Whole length of mylohyoid line of mandible	Body of hyoid bone	▲ hyoid & tongue	Mylohyoid n.	Lingual a.
Geniohyoideus	Inf mental spine on inner surface of -symphysis menti	Ant surface of hyoid	Draws hyoid & tongue ant	1st cervical n. (through hypoglossal n.)	Lingual a.
Infrahyoid Group					
Sternohyoideus	Post surface of med end of clavicle, post sternoclav lig & sup & post part of manubrium sterni	Inf border of hyoid bone	Draws hyoid inferiorly	Branch of ansa cervicalis (1st three cervical nerves)	Lingual a. Subclavian a.
Sternothyroideus	Dorsal surface of manubrium sterni (caudal of origin of sternohyoideus)	Oblique line on lamina of thyroid cartilage	Draws thyroid caudally	Branch of ansa cervicalis (1st three cervical nerves)	Lingual a. Subclavian a.
Thyrohyoideus	Oblique line on lamina of thyroid cartilage	Inf border of greater cornu of hyoid bone	Draws hyoid inferiorly Draws thyroid cartilage sup	1st & 2nd cervical n.	Lingual a. Subclavian a.
Omohyoideus	Cranial border of scapula (near or crossing scapular notch)	Caudal border of hyoid bone	Draws hyoid caudally	Branch of ansa cervicalis (1st three cervical nerves)	Subclavian a.

Neck

Muscle	Origin	Insertion	Action	Nerve	Artery
Longus Colli	Vertical: ant surface of C5, C6, C7, T1, T2 & T3; Sup: ant tubercles of transverse processes C3, C4, C5; Inf: ant surface of T2 & T3	Vertical: ant surface of C2, C3, C4; Sup: narrow tendon into tubercle on ant arch of atlas; Inf: ant tubercles of transverse processes C5 & C6	✓ neck ↻ neck (min)	Branches of 2nd to 7th cervical nerves	Subclavian a. (thyrocervical)
Longus Capitus	Four tendinous slips from ant tubercles of transverse processes C3, C4, C5 & C6	Inf surface of the basilar part of occipital bone	Head ✓	Branches from 1st, 2nd, & 3rd cervical nerves	Subclavian a.
Rectus Capitus Anterior	Ant surface of lat mass of the atlas & from root of its transverse process	Inf surface of basilar part of occipital bone	Head ✓	Branch of 1st & 2nd cervical nerves	Subclavian a.
Rectus Capitus Lateralis	Sup surface of transverse process of atlas	Inf surface of jugular process of occipital bone	Lat ✓ head	Branch of 1st & 2nd cervical nerves	Subclavian a.
Scalenus Anterior	Ant tubercles of transverse processes of C3, C4, C5 & C6	Scalene tubercle on inner border of 1st rib & ridge on cranial surface of rib	▲ 1st rib ✓ head ↻ head	Branches of lower cervical nerves	Subclavian a. (thyrocervical)

Muslce	Origin	Insertion	Action	Nerve	Artery
Neck					
Scalenus Medius	Post tubercles of transverse processes of C2, C3, C4, C5, C6 & C7	Cranial surface of 1st rib between tubercle & subclavian groove	◂ 1st rib ↙ head ↻ head	Branches from cervical nerves	Subclavian a. (thyrocervical)
Scalenus Posterior	Post tubercles of transverse processes of C5, C6 & C7	Outer surface of 2nd rib (deep to serratus anterior)	◂ 2nd rib ↙ head ↻ head	Ventral primary branches C5, C6 & C7	Subclavian a.
Back/Neck					
Serratus Posterior Superior	Caudal part of ligamentum nuchae, spinous processes C7, T1, T2 & T3; supraspinal ligament	Four digitations—cranial borders of ribs 2, 3, 4 & 5	Respiratory ◂ ribs	Ventral rami T1-T4	Subclavian a.
Serratus Posterior Inferior	Spinous processes T11, T12, L1, L2 & L3; supraspinal ligament	Four digitations into inf borders last 4 ribs (a little beyond their angles)	Respiratory Draws ribs ◂▸ & ▾	Ventral rami T9-T12	Subclavian a.
Splenius Capitis Cervicis	Caudal ½ ligamentum nuchae & spinous processes C7, T1, T2, T3 & sometimes T4	Occipital bone just inf to lat 1/3 of sup nuchal line; into mastoid process of temporal bone	↙ head & neck lat ✓ same side ↻ same side	Lat branches dorsal primary cervical nerves	Subclavian a. (branches)

Back/Neck

Muscle	Origin	Insertion	Action	Nerve	Artery
Spinalis Capitis	Usually inseparable from semispinalis capitis		/ spine	Branch dorsal primary spinal nerves	Thoracic aorta (branch)
Semispinalis Capitis	Tips of transverse processes C7, T1, T2, T3, T4, T5, T6 & sometimes T7	Between sup & inf nuchal lines of occipital bone	/ head & neck ↻ opp side	Dorsal rami	Subclavian a. (branches)
Longissimus Capitis	Transverse processes T4 & T5 and cervicis & articular processes C4 C5, C6 & C7	Post margin of mastoid process (deep to splenius capitis & SCM)	/ head ↻ same side ↙ same side	Dorsal primary mid & lower cervical n(s).	Subclavian a. (branches)
Obliquus Capitis Inferior	Arises from apex of spinous process of axis	Inf & dorsal transverse process of atlas	↻ same side	Branch dorsal primary division suboccipital n.	Subclavian a. (branch)
Obliquus Capitis Superior	Tendinous fibers from sup surface transverse process of atlas	Occipital bone between sup & inf nuchal lines (lat to semispinalis capitis)	/ head	Branch dorsal primary division suboccipital n.	Subclavian a. (branch)
Rectus Capitis Posterior Major	Spinous process of the axis	Lat part of inf nuchal line of occipital bone and surface immediately inf	/ head ↻ same side	Branch dorsal primary division suboccipital n.	Subclavian a. (branch)

Muscle	Origin	Insertion	Action	Nerve	Artery
Back/Neck					
Rectus Capitis Posterior Minor	Tendon from tubercle on post arch of atlas	Med part of the inf nuchal line of occipital bone & surface between it & foramen magnum	/ head	Branch dorsal primary division suboccipital n.	Subclavian a. (branch)
Longissimus Cervicis	Long thin tendons from apex transverse processes upper 4 or 5 thoracic vertebrae	Post tubercles of transverse processes of C2-C6	/ spine lat ✓ ▶ ribs	Dorsal primary branch spinal nerves	Branches thoracic aorta
Iliocostalis Cervicis	Angles of the 3rd, 4th, 5th & 6th ribs	Post tubercles of transverse processes of C4, C5 & C6	/ spine lat ✓ ▶ ribs	Dorsal primary branch spinal nerves	Thoracic aorta (branches)
Spinalis Cervicis	Caudal part of ligamentum nuchae, spinous process C7; sometimes T1 & T2	Spinous processes of axis; sometimes spinous process C1 & C2	/ spine	Dorsal primary branch spinal nerves	Thoracic aorta (branch)
Semispinalis Cervicis	Transverse processes of 1st five or six thoracic vertebrae	Cervical spinous processes from axis to C5	/ spine ↻ opp side	Dorsal primary branch spinal nerves	Thoracic aorta (branch)

Muscle	Origin	Insertion	Action	Nerve	Artery
Back					
Longissimus Thoracis	Arising from erector spinae & post surfaces transverse & accessory processes of lumbar vertebrae & ant layer lumbocostal aponeurosis	Transverse processes of all thoracic vertebrae and lower 9 or 10 ribs between tubercles and angles	/ spine lat ✓ ▼ ribs	Dorsal primary branch spinal nerves	Thoracic aorta (branch)
Iliocostalis Thoracis	Flattened tendons from upper borders of angles of lower 6 ribs (med to iliocostalis lumborum)	Cranial borders of angles of 1st 6 ribs and into dorsum of transverse process C7	/ spine lat ✓ ▼ ribs	Dorsal primary branch spinal nerves	Thoracic aorta (branch)
Spinalis Thoracis	Med continuation of sacrospinalis. Arises from spinous processes of T11, T12, L1 & L2	Spinous processes of upper thoracic vertebrae	/ spine	Dorsal primary branch spinal nerves	Thoracic aorta (branch)
Semispinalis Thoracis	Transverse processes of T6-T10	Spinous processes of C6, C7, T1, T2, T3 & T4	/ spine ↻ opp side	Dorsal primary branch spinal nerves	Thoracic aorta (branch)
Iliocostalis Lumborum	Flattened tendons from upper portion of erector	Inf borders of angles of last 6 or 7 ribs	/ spine lat ✓ ▼ ribs	Dorsal primary branch spinal nerves	Thoracic aorta (branch)

Muscle	Origin	Insertion	Action	Nerve	Artery
Back					
Sacrospinalis (Erector Spinae)	Arises from broad tendon attached to mid crest of sacrum; spinous processes T11-T12 & lumbar vertebrae; supraspinal ligament to lip of iliac crests & lat crest of sacrum	Splits into longissimus, iliocostalis, spinalis, & semispinalis muscles (see respective muscles)	/ spine ↻ spine ▼ ribs lat ✓	Spinal nerves	Thoracic aorta
Multifidus	Spinous processes of each vertebra from sacrum to axis; arises from back of sacrum from aponeurosis of sacrospinalis, from med surface of post sup iliac spine & post sacroiliac ligaments	Each ascends obliquely crossing over 2-4 vertebrae and inserted into spinous process of vertebra from last lumbar to axis	/ spine ↻ opp side	Branches of dorsal primary spinal nerves	Thoracic aorta
Rotatores	Transverse process of one vertebra & insert at base of spinous process of vertebra above from the sacrum to the axis	*Rotatores longi* cross one vertebra in their oblique course. *Rotatores breves* insert in next succeeding vertebra & run horizontal	/ spine ↻ opp side	Branches of dorsal primary spinal nerves	Thoracic aorta

Muscle	Origin	Insertion	Action	Nerve	Artery
Back					
Quadratus Lumborum	Sup borders of the transverse processes L2-L5	Inf border of last rib & transverse process L1-L4	▼ last rib; lat ✓	12th thoracic n. 1st lumbar n.	Iliac circumflex
Shoulder Girdle					
Trapezius	Ext occipital protuberance; med 1/3 sup nuchal line; spinous process C7, T1-T12	Post border of lat 3rd clavicle; med margin acromion; spine of the scapula	▲ &r/shoulder; Abd same side; ↻ opp side; Retraction; ▲ ↻ glen fossa	Spinal accessory n. C3 & C4 spinal nerves	Suprascapular
Levator Scapulae	Transverse processes C1-C4	Med border scapula between sup angle & spine	Elevation; Protraction / cervical spine; Abd same side; ↻ glen fossa	Dorsal scapular n. C3 & C4 spinal nerves	Superficial cervical a. Transverse cervical a.
Romboideus Minor	Spinous process of C7 & T1	Med border scapula at level of the spine	Elevation; Retraction; ▼ ↻ glen fossa	Dorsal scapular n.	Descending scapular a.
Romboideus Major	Spinous process of T2-T5	Med border scapula between spine & inf angle	Elevation; Retraction; ▼ ↻ glen fossa	Dorsal scapular n.	Descending scapular a.

Muscle	Origin	Insertion	Action	Nerve	Artery
Shoulder Girdle					
Latissimus Dorsi	Lumbar aponeurosis; spinous processes of T6-T12, L1-L5 & sacral vertebrae	Distal part of intertubercular groove of humerus	/ shoulder Abd shoulder Med ↻ Elevation Retraction	Thoracodorsal n. C6-C8 spinal nerves	Subscapular a.
Pectoralis Major	Ant surface sternal 1/2 clavicle; ventral surface sternum; aponeurosis of obliquus externus abdominis	Crest of greater tubercle of humerus	✓ shoulder Add shoulder Med ↻ Protract; ▲▼	Med & lat pectoral n. C5-C8 spinal nerves 1st thoracic n.	Thoraco-acromial a.
Pectoralis Minor	Ext surfaces of ribs 3, 4 & 5 near their cartilages	Caracoid process of scapula	Protraction Depression ▼↻ glen fossa	Med pectoral n.	Thoraco-acromial a.
Subclavius	1st rib & its cartilage near their junction	Inf aspect of clavicle in the mid 3rd	Protraction Depression	Branch from brachial plexus (sup trunk)	Thoraco-acromial a.
Serratus Anterior	Ext surfaces of ribs 1-9	Ant aspect of med border of scapula from sup to inf angle	Protraction Depression ◄↻ glen fossa	Long thoracic n.	Lat thoracic a.
Subscapularis	Mid 2/3 subscapular fossa; inf 2/3 groove on axillary	Lesser tubercle of humerus	Med ↻ ✓ & / Abd & add	Subscapular n.	Circumflex scapular a.

Muscle	Origin	Insertion	Action	Nerve	Artery
Shoulder Girdle					
Supraspinatus	Mid 2/3 supraspina-tous fossa	Sub impression of greater tubercle of humerus	Abd Lat ↻(weak) ✓ (weak)	Suprascapular n.	Suprascapular a.
Infraspinatus	Med 2/3 infraspinatus fossa	Mid impression of greater tubercle of humerus	Lat ↻ Abd & add	Suprascapular n.	Suprascapular a.
Teres Minor	Dorsal surface of axillary border of scapula	Inf impression of greater tubercle of humerus distal to inf impression	Lat ↻ Add	Branch of axillary n.	Post humeral circumflex a.
Teres Major	Oval area on dorsal surface of inf angle of scapula	Crest of lesser tubercle of humerus	Add / shoulder Med ↻	Lower subscapular n.	Circumflex scapular a.
Deltoideus surface of lat 3rd of -	Ant border & sup clavicle; lat margin & sup surface of acromium; inf lip post border scapular spine	Deltoid prominence on mid of lat body of humerus	Abd shoulder / shoulder / shoulder Med & lat ↻	Axillary n. from brachial plexus	Post humeral circumflex a.
Shoulder/Elbow					
Triceps Brachii	Long head: infraglenoid tuberosity of scapula;	Post proximal surface of olecranon	/ elbow / shoulder	Branches radial n.	Profunda brachii a.

Muscle	Origin	Insertion	Action	Nerve	Artery
Shoulder/Elbow					
Brachialis	Lat head: post surface of humerus; Med head: post surface of humerus distal to radial groove	Tuberosity of ulna; rough depression on ant surface of coronoid process	Add shoulder		Inf ulnar collateral a.
Biceps Brachii	Distal 1/2 of ant-aspect of humerus	Rough post portion tuberosity of radius	✓elbow	Musculocutaneous n. Radial & med n.	Brachial a.
Coracobrachialis	Short head: apex of coracoid process; Long head: supraglenoid tuberosity at sup margin of glenoid	Impression at med surface & border of humerus	✓ shoulder ✓ elbow Supination	Musculocutaneous n.	Brachial a.
	Apex of coracoid process		✓ shoulder Add shoulder	Musculocutaneous n.	Brachial a.
Forearm/Wrist					
Pronator Teres	Humeral head: proximal to med epicondyle of humerus; Ulnar head: med side of coronoid process of ulna	Rough impression at mid of lat surface of radius	Pronation	Median n.	Inf ulnar collateral a.

Forearm/Wrist

Muscle	Origin	Insertion	Action	Nerve	Artery
Flexor Carpi Radialis	Med epicondyle of humerus	Base of 2nd metacarpal bone	✓ wrist, Radial ✓	Median n.	Radial a.
Palmaris Longus	Med epicondyle of humerus	Palmar aponeurosis	✓ wrist	Median n.	Volar interosseous a.
Flexor Carpi Ulnaris	Humeral head: med epicondyle of humerus; Ulnar head: med margin olecranon; proximal 2/3 dorsal border of ulna	Pisiform bone	✓ wrist, Add wrist	Ulnar n.	Ulnar a.
Flexor Digitorum Superficialis	Humeral head: med epicondyle of humerus; Ulnar head: med side of coronoid process; Radial head: oblique line of radius	Divides into 4 tendons which are inserted into the sides of the 2nd phalanx	✓ PIPs, ✓ MCPs, ✓ wrist	Median n.	Ulnar a.
Flexor Digitorum Profundus	Proximal 3/4 of volar & med surfaces of body of ulnar	Bases of last phalanges	✓ DIPs, ✓ PIPs, ✓ MCPs, ✓ wrist	Palmar interosseous n. from median n. Branch of ulnar n.	Ulnar a., Volar interosseous a.
Flexor Pollicis Longus	Grooved volar surface of body of the radius	Base of distal phalanx of the thumb	✓ IP digit I, ✓ MCP digit I, ✓ & add wrist	Palmar interosseous n. from median n.	Radial a.

Muscle	Origin	Insertion	Action	Nerve	Artery
Forearm/Wrist					
Pronator Quadratus	Pronator ridge on distal part of palmar surface of body of ulna; med part of palmar surface of distal 1/4 of ulna	Distal 1/4 of lat border & palmar surface of body of the radius	Pronation	Palmar interosseous n. from median n.	Ulnar & radial a.
Brachioradialis	Proximal 2/3 of lat supracondylar ridge of humerus	Lat side of base of styloid process of radius	✓ elbow	Branch of radial n.	Radial a.
Extensor Carpi Radialis Longus	Distal 1/3 lat supracondylar ridge of humerus	Dorsal surface of base of 2nd metacarpal bone—radial side	/ extension Abd wrist	Radial n.	Radial a.
Extensor Carpi Radialis Brevis	Lat epicondyle of humerus	Dorsal surface of base of 3rd metacarpal bone—radial side	/ wrist Abd wrist	Radial n.	Radial a.
Extensor Carpi Ulnaris	Lat epicondyle of humerus	Prominent tubercle on ulnar side of base of metacarpal V	/ wrist Add wrist	Deep radial n.	Ulnar a.
Extensor Digitorum	Lat epicondyle of humerus	2nd & 3rd phalanges of fingers; dorsal surface of distal phalanx	/ PIPs & DIPs; / MCPs / wrist	Deep radial n.	Ulnar a.
Extensor Digiti Minimi	Common extensor tendon	Expansion of ext digitorum tendon on dorsum of 1st phalanx of little finger	/ PIPs, DIPs & MCP digit V	Deep radial n.	Ulnar a.

Muscle	Origin	Insertion	Action	Nerve	Artery
Forearm/Wrist					
Anconeus	Separate tendon from dorsal part of lat epicondyle of humerus	Side of olecranon; proximal 1/4 of dorsal surface of body of ulna	/ elbow	Radial n.	Ulnar a.
Abductor Pollicis Longus	Lat part of dorsal surface of body of ulna	Radial side of base of 1st metacarpal bone	Abd IP, MCP of digit I Abd wrist	Deep radial n.	Radial a.
Extensor Pollicis Brevis	Dorsal surface of body of radius distal to that muscle & interosseous membrane	Base of 1st phalanx of thumb	/ IP, MCP of digit I / wrist	Deep radial n.	Radial a.
Extensor Pollicis Longus	Lat part of mid 1/3 of dorsal surface of body of ulna distal to origin of abductor pollicis longus	Base of last phalanx of thumb	/ IP, MCP of digit I / wrist	Deep radial n.	Radial a.
Extensor Indicis	Dorsal surface of body of ulna below origin of extensor pollicis longus	Joins ulnar side of - tendon of extensor - digitorum	/ & add of IP, MCP digit II	Deep radial n.	Radial a.
Supinator	Lat epicondyle of humerus from ridge of ulna	Lat edge of radial tuberosity & oblique line of radius & med surface of radius posteriorly	Supination	Deep radial n.	Radial a.

Muscle	Origin	Insertion	Action	Nerve	Artery
Hand					
Abductor Pollicis Brevis	Transverse carpal ligament, tuberosity of scaphoid, ridge of trapezium	Radial side of base of 1st phalanx thumb	Abd thumb	Median n.	Radial a.
Opponens Pollicis	Ridge of trapezium	Length of metacarpal bone of thumb on radial side	Abd thumb ✓ thumb Med ↻	Median n.	Radial a.
Flexor Pollicis Brevis	Distal ridge of trapezium; ulnar side of 1st metacarpal	Radial side of base of proximal phalanx of thumb; ulnar side of base of 1st phalanx	✓ thumb Add thumb	Median & ulnar n.	Radial a.
Adductor Pollicis	Capitate bone, bases of 2nd & 3rd metacarpals	Ulnar side of base of proximal phalanx of thumb	Add thumb	Deep palmar branch of ulnar n.	Ulnar n.
Palmaris Brevis	Tendinous fasciculi from palmar aponeurosis	Skin on ulnar border of palm of hand	Draws skin mid palm	Ulnar n.	Superficial ulnar a.
Abductor Digiti Minimi	Pisiform bone	Ulnar side of base of 1st phalanx of digit V	Abd digit V ✓ proximal phalanx	Ulnar n.	Ulnar a.
Flexor Digiti Minimi Brevis	Convex surface of hamulus of hamate bone	Ulnar side of base of 1st phalanx of digit V	✓ digit V	Ulnar n.	Ulnar a.

Muscle	Origin	Insertion	Action	Nerve	Artery
Hand					
Opponens Digiti Minimi	Convexity of hamulus of hamate bone	Length of metacarpal bone of digit V along ulnar margin	Abd digit V ↓ digit V Med ↓ V	Ulnar n.	Ulnar a.
Lumbricals	Originate from the profundus tendons. 1 & 2: radials sides & palmar surfaces of tendons of digits II & III; 3: contiguous sides of mid & ring fingers; 4: contiguous sides of tendons of ring & little finger	Tendinous expansion of extensor digitorum	✓ MCPs / PIPs & DIPs	1 & 2: median n. 3 & 4: ulnar n.	Median a. Ulnar a.
Interosseous Dorsales Interossei	Two heads from adjacent sides of metacarpal bone; all from entire length of metacarpal bones	Bases of 1st phalanx; Side of base of 1st phalanx	Abd—midline (digit III) ✓ MCPs / PIPs & DIPs; Add—midline (digit III)	Deep palmar (digit III); Deep palmar branch n.	Ulnar a. branch n.; Ulnar a.
Hip					
Psoas Major (Iliopsoas)	Ventral surface of bases and caudal borders of transverse process of	Lesser trochanter of femur	✓ hip ✓ spine in lumbar region	2nd & 3rd lumbar n	Lumbar branch of iliolumbar a.

Muscle	Origin	Insertion	Action	Nerve	Artery
Hip					
	lumbar spine; sides and corresponding intervertebral disks of last thoracic and all lumbar vertebrae				
Psoas Minor (Iliopsoas)	Vertebral margins of T12 & L1, & corresponding disks	Pectineal line; iliopectineal eminence	✓ spine in lumbar region	1st & 2nd lumbar n.	Lumbar branch of iliolumbar a.
Iliacus (Iliopsoas)	Upper 2/3 of iliac fossa; iliac crest	Lesser trochanter of femur	✓ at hip	Femoral n. (muscular branches)	Lumbar branch of iliolumbar a.
Tensor Fasciae Latae (TFL)	Ant part of outer lip of iliac crest, ant border of ilium	Lat part of fascia lata at junction of proximal & mid thirds of thigh (proximal end of iliotibial band)	Tenses TFL ✓ at hip Abd at hip Int ↻ at hip	Sup gluteal n.	Sup gluteal a.
Gluteus Maximus	Post gluteal line; dorsal surface of sacrum & coccyx	Gluteal tuberosity; lat part of TFL at junction of proximal and mid thirds of thigh (proximal end of iliotibial band)	/ at hip Add at hip Ext ↻ at hip / lower spine	Inf gluteal n.	Inf gluteal a.

Muscle **Hip**	Origin	Insertion	Action	Nerve	Artery
Gluteus Medius	Outer surface of ilium from iliac crest & post gluteal line above to ant gluteal line below	Lat surface of greater trochanter	Abd at hip Int ↻ at hip	Sup gluteal n.	Sup gluteal a.
Piriformis	Pelvic surface of sacrum between ant sacral foramina & margin of greater sciatic foramen	Upper border of greater trochanter of femur	Ext ↻ at hip Abd at hip	1st & 2nd sacral n.	Sup gluteal a.
Obturator Internus	Margins of obturator foramen; pelvic surface of hip bone; post & sup obturator foramen	Med surface of greater trochanter	Ext ↻ at hip Abd at hip	Obturator n. to obturator internus & gemellus sup	Obturator a. Sup gluteal a.
Gemellus Superior	Outer surface of ischial spine	Med surface of greater trochanter	Ext ↻ at hip	Obturator n. to obturator internus & gemellus sup	Obturator a. Sup gluteal a.
Gemellus Inferior	Upper part of ischial tuberosity	Med surface of greater trochanter	Ext ↻ at hip	Obturator n. to quadratus femoris & gemellus inf	Sup gluteal a.
Quadratus Femoris	Lat margin of ischial tuberosity	Quadrate tubercle of femur; linea quadrata	Add at hip Ext ↻ at hip	Obturator n. to quadratus femoris & gemellus inf	Sup gluteal a.
Obturator Externus	Outer margin of obturator foramen	Trochanteric fossa of femur	Add at hip Ext ↻ at hip	Post branch of obturator n.	Obturator a.

Muscle	Origin	Insertion	Action	Nerve	Artery
Hip/Thigh					
Sartorius	Ant-sup iliac spine; upper half of iliac notch	Upper part of med surface of tibia	✓ at hip, Ext↻ at knee, ✓ at knee, Abd hip (weak)	Muscular branches of femoral n.	Femoral a.
Quadriceps Femoris					
Rectus Femoris	Ant-inf iliac spine	Patella by the patellar ligament to the tibial tuberosity	✓ at knee, ✓ at hip	Muscular branches of femoral n.	Femoral a.
Vastus Lateralis	Lat aspect of the shaft of the femur	Patella by the patellar ligament to the tibial tuberosity	✓ at knee	Muscular branches of femoral n.	Femoral a.
Vastus Medialis	Med aspect of the shaft of the femur	Patella by the patellar ligament to the tibial tuberosity	✓ at knee, draws patella medially	Muscular branches of femoral n.	Femoral a.
Vastus Intermedius	Ant aspect of the shaft of the femur	Patella by the patellar ligament to the tibial tuberosity	✓ at knee	Muscular branches of femoral n.	Femoral a.
Gracilis	Lower 1/2 of pubic symphysis; upper 1/2 of pubic arch	Proximal part of med surface of tibia	✓ at knee, Int↻ at knee, Add at hip	Ant branch of obturator n.	Med femoral circumflex a. (ascending)
Pectineus	Pubic pectineal line & an area of bone ant to it	Line leading from the lesser trochanter to the linea aspera	Add at hip, ✓ at hip, Int↻ hip	Muscular branches of femoral & obturator n.	Med femoral circumflex a.

Hip/Thigh

Muscle	Origin	Insertion	Action	Nerve	Artery
Adductor Longus	Ant portion of pubis in angle between crest & symphysis	Mid part of linea aspera	Add at hip / ✓ at hip	Ant branch of obturator n.	Profunda femoris a.
Adductor Brevis	Ext surface of inf ramus of pubis	Proximal part of linea aspera	Add at hip / ✓ at hip	Ant branch of obturator n.	Mid femoral circumflex a.
Adductor Magnus	Pubic arch & ischial tuberosity	Oblique line along entire shaft of the femur	Add at hip / ✓ hip (upper) / hip (lower)	Post branch of obturator & sciatic n.	Profunda femoris & med femoris circumflex a.
Biceps Femoris	Long head: from ischial tuberosity; Short head: lat lip of linea aspera; lat supra-condylar line of femur	Head of fibula, lat condyle of tibia, deep fascia on lat side of leg	✓ at knee / at hip / Ext ↻ knee (semiflexed)	Sciatic n. tibial branch to long head; peroneal branch to short head	Profunda femoris a.
Semitendinous	Upper & mid impression of ischial tuberosity (with tendon of the biceps femoris)	Proximal part of ant border & med surface of the tibia	✓ at knee / at hip / Int ↻ knee (semiflexed)	Sciatic n.	Perforating branch profunda femoris a.
Semimembranous	Proximal & lat facet of ischial tuberosity	Med-post surface of med condyle of tibia	✓ at knee / at hip / Int ↻ knee (semiflexed)	Sciatic n.	Perforating branch profunda femoris a.

Muscle	Origin	Insertion	Action	Nerve	Artery
Leg					
Tibialis Anterior	Lat surface of shaft of tibia; med aspect of fibula; ant interosseous membrane	Med & plantar surface of med cuniform bone; base of 1st metatarsal bone	Dorsiflexion inversion	Deep peroneal n.	Ant tibial a.
Popliteus	Lat condyle of femur	Triangular area on post surface of tibia above sdeal line	✓ at knee Int ↻ at knee	Tibial n. (med & int popliteal)	Post tibial a.
Leg/Foot					
Extensor Hallucis Longus	Lat surface of shaft of tibia; med aspect of fibula; ant interosseous membrane	Base of distal phalanx of great toe	/ MTP & IP Dorsiflexion	Deep peroneal n. (ant tibial)	Ant tibial a.
Extensor Digitorum Longus (EDL)	Lat surface of shaft of tibia; med aspect of fibula; ant - interosseous membrane	Dorsal surface of mid & distal phalanges of lat 4 digits	/ IPs digits II to V Dorsiflexion	Deep peroneal n. (ant tibial)	Ant tibial a.
Extensor Digitorum Brevis (EDB)	Proximal & lat surface of calcaneus; lat talo-calcaneal ligament	1st tendon dorsal surface of base of proximal phalanx of hallux; other 3 tendons lat sides of tendons of EDL	/ IPs	Deep peroneal n.	Ant tibial a.

Muscle	Origin	Insertion	Action	Nerve	Artery
Leg/Foot					
Flexor Digitorum Longus	Post surface of shaft of tibia; post aspect of fibula; post interosseous membrane	Plantar surface of base of distal phalanx lat 4 digits	✓ digits II to V Plantar-flexion	Tibial n. (med & int popliteal)	Post tibial a.
Flexor Hallucis Longus	Post surface of shaft of tibia; post aspect of fibula; post interosseous membrane	Base of distal phalanx of hallux	✓ digit I Plantarflexion	Tibial n. (med & int popliteal)	Post tibial a.
Tibialis Posterior	Post surface of shaft of tibia; post aspect of fibula; ant interosseous membrane	Tuberosity of navicular; plantar surface of cuniform bones; plantar surface of base of 2nd, 3rd & 4th metatarsals, cuboid, sustentaculum tali	Plantarflexion Inversion	Tibial n. (med & int popliteal)	Post tibial a.
Peroneus Tertius	Lat surface of shaft of tibia; med aspect of fibula; ant interosseous membrane	Dorsal surface of base of 5th metatarsal bone	Dorsiflexion Eversion	Deep peroneal n. (ant tibial)	Ant tibial a.
Peroneus Longus	Lat condyle of tibia; head & upper 2/3 of lat surface of fibula	Lat side of med cuniform bone, base of 1st metatarsal bone	Plantarflexion Eversion	Superficial peroneal n. (musculocutaneous)	Peroneal a.

Muscle	Origin	Insertion	Action	Nerve	Artery
Leg/Foot					
Peroneus Brevis	Lower 2/3 of lat surface of fibula	Lat side of base of 5th metatarsal bone	Plantarflexion Eversion	Superficial peroneal n. (musculocutaneous)	Peroneal a.
Gastrocnemius	Med head: med condyle & adjacent part of femur; capsule of knee; Long head: lat condyle & adjacent part of femur; capsule of knee	Calcaneus by the calcaneal tendon	Plantarflexion ✓ at knee	Tibial n. (med popliteal)	Popliteal a.
Soleus	Post surface of head & proximal 1/3 of shaft of fibula; mid 1/3 of med border of tibia	Calcaneus by the calcaneal tendon	Plantarflexion	Tibial n. (med popliteal)	Post tibial a.
Plantaris	Lat supracondylar line of femur	Med side of post part of calcaneus	Plantarflexion	Tibial n. (med popliteal)	Post tibial a.
Foot					
Quadratus Plantae	Med head: med surface of calcaneus & med border of long plantar ligament; Lat head: lat border of plantar surface of calcaneus & lat border of long plantar ligament	Attached to tendons of flexor digitorum longus	✓ last IP digits II to V	Lat plantar n.	Lat plantar a.

Muscle	Origin	Insertion	Action	Nerve	Artery
Foot					
Lumbricals (4)	Tendons of flexor digitorum longus	Tendons of EDL & interossei into bases of last phalanges of digits II-V	✓ MP joints / IP joints	Med plantar n. Deep lat plantar n.	Med plantar a.

Key:
✓ flexion
/ extension
↻ rotation
▼ depression, downward, caudal
▲ elevation, upward, cephalic
◄► outward, expand
n. = nerve
a. = artery
Lat = lateral
Med = medial
Ext = external
Int = internal
Sup = superior
Inf = inferior

Ant = anterior
Post = posterior
Min = minimal
MTP = metatarsophalangeal
MCP = metacarpophalangeal
IP = interphalangeal
PIP = proximal interphalangeal
DIP = distal interphalangeal
Opp = opposite
Abd = abduction
Add = adduction
Mid = middle

Reprinted with permission from Bottomley J. *Quick Reference Dictionary for Physical Therapy*. Thorofare, NJ: SLACK Incorporated; 2000.

APPENDIX 6

Normal Joint Ranges of Motion

Cervical Spine

Flexion	0 to (45-90°)
Extension	0 to (50-70°)
Lateral flexion	0 to (20-45°)
Rotation	0 to (60-90°)

Lumbar Spine

Flexion	0 to (40-60°)
Extension	0 to (20-35°)
Lateral flexion	0 to (15-20°)
Rotation	0 to (3-12°)

Shoulder

Flexion	0 to (167-180°)
Extension	0 to (45-62°)
Abduction	0 to (170-184°)
Internal rotation	0 to (69-90°)
External rotation	0 to (90-104°)
Horizontal flexion (adduction)	0 to (30-45°)
Horizontal extension (abduction)	0 to (135-140°)

Elbow

Flexion	0 to (135-150°)
Pronation	0 to (75-90°)
Supination	0 to (70-90°)

Wrist

Flexion	0 to (60-90°)
Extension	0 to (50-90°)
Abduction	0 to (40-45°)
Adduction	0 to (15-30°)

Hand

Fingers 2-5
    MCP
        Flexion   0 to (85-90°)
        Extension   0 to (30-45°)
    PIP
        Flexion   0 to (100-115°)
        Extension   0°
    DIP
        Flexion   0 to (80-90°)
        Extension   0 to 20°
        Abduction   0 to (20-30°)
Thumb
    CM
        Flexion   0 to 50°
        Extension   0°
    MCP
        Flexion   0 to 55°
        Extension   0°
    IP
        Flexion   0 to 90°
        Extension   0 to 5°
        Abduction   0 to 70°
        Adduction   0 to 30°

Hip

Flexion	0 to (100-130°)
Extension	0 to (15-50°)
Abduction	0 to (40-50°)

Adduction	0 to (15-45°)
Internal rotation	0 to (30-45°)
External rotation	0 to (35-50°)
Horizontal flexion (adduction)	0 to 40°
Horizontal extension (abduction)	0 to (50-90°)

Knee

Flexion	0 to (120-145°)

Ankle

Plantar flexion	0 to (40-65°)
Dorsiflexion	0 to (10-30°)
Inversion	0 to (30-50°)
Eversion	0 to (15-25°)
Supination	0 to (45-60°)
Pronation	0 to (20-30°)

Foot

MTP flexion (great toe)	0 to 45°
MTP flexion (toes 2-5)	0 to 40°
MTP extension (great toe)	0 to 70°
MTP extension (toes 2-5)	0 to 40°
IP flexion (great toe)	0 to 90°
IP extension (great toe)	0°
DIP flexion (toes 2-5)	0 to 60°
PIP flexion (toes 2-5)	0 to 35°
DIP extension (toes 2-5)	0 to 30°
PIP extension (toes 2-5)	0°

APPENDIX 7

Cranial Nerves

I	Olfactory	Smell
II	Optic	Visual acuity, reaction to light
III	Oculomotor	Blinking/eye movement
IV	Trochlear	Inferiolateral eye movement
V	Trigeminal	Facial sensation
VI	Abducens	Lateral eye movement
VII	Facial	Facial movements, scrunch face, pout, smile, taste
VIII	Vestibulocochlear	Hearing/balance
IX	Glossopharyngeal	Taste, tongue movements
X	Vagus	Breathing, taste, swallowing
XI	Accessory	Neck flexion, shrug shoulders
XII	Hypoglosseal	Tongue movements

APPENDIX 8

Comparison of Concussions Grading Systems

Grade	Cantu	Colorado	AAN
Grade 1	no LOC amnesia <30 min	no LOC amnesia <30 min	concussion symptoms <15 min, no amnesia
Grade 2	LOC <5 min amnesia >30 min	LOC <5 min amnesia >30 min	concussion symptoms >15 min
Grade 3	LOC >5 min amnesia >24 hr	any loss of consciousness	any loss of consciousness

Comparison of Return to Play Guidelines

Grade	Cantu	Colorado	AAN
Grade 1			
1st concussion	When asymptomatic	Asymptomatic for 20 min	Asymptomatic for 15 min
2nd concussion	2 weeks when asymptomatic for 1 week	When asymptomatic for 1 week	When asymptomatic for 1 week
3rd concussion	Terminate season	May return in 3 months	—
Grade 2			
1st concussion	When asymptomatic for 1 week	When asymptomatic for 1 week	When asymptomatic for 1 week
2nd concussion	1 month consider termination	When asymptomatic for 1 month	When asymptomatic for 2 weeks
3rd concussion	—	—	—
Grade 3			
1st concussion	1 month when asymptomatic for 1 week	Immediate referral, return 1 month if asymptomatic for 2 weeks	Immediate referral, return when asymptomatic for 1 week
2nd concussion	Terminate season	Terminate season	When asymptomatic for 1 month
3rd concussion	—	—	—

AAN = American Academy of Neurology; LOC = Loss of consciousness

Adapted from Harmon KG. *Assessment and management of concussion in sports.* Am Fam Physician. 1999;60;887-94. Available at: www.aafp.org/afp/990901ap/887.html. Accessed 2001.

APPENDIX 9

Nerve Root Assessment—Upper Extremity

Nerve Root	Dermatome	Myotome	Reflex
C4	Top shoulder and neck	Elevate shoulders	—
C5	Lateral upper arm, shoulder	Shoulder abduction	Biceps
C6	Later arm, thumb	Elbow flexion/ wrist extension	Brachioradialis
C7	Middle finger, posterior middle arm	Elbow extension/ wrist flexion	Triceps
C8	Medial hand	Finger flexion	—
T1	Medial elbow	Finger abduction/ adduction	—

Appendix 10

Nerve Root Assessment—Lower Extremity

Nerve Root	Dermatome	Myotome	Reflex
L1	Anterior upper thigh, lateral hip	Hip flexion	—
L2	Anterior mid thigh	Hip flexion, knee extension	Patella
L3	Lower anterior medial thigh (area of vastus medialis oblique [vmol])	Knee extension	Patella
L4	Anterior/medial leg	Dorsiflexion (heel walking)	Patella
L5	Anterior/lateral leg	Knee flexion, great toe extension	Tibialis posterior
S1	Lateral ankle	Knee flexion, plantar-flexion (toe walking)	Achilles'
S2	Posterior superior lower leg	—	—

APPENDIX 11

Peripheral Nerve Innervations—Upper Extremity

Peripheral Nerve	Sensory Area	Manual Muscle Test (see Figures 1 and 2 for complete list)
Axillary (C5-6)	Upper deltoid area	Deltoid, teres minor
Musculocutaneous (C5-7)	Anterior and lateral upper arm	Biceps brachii
Radial (C5-T1)	Posterior arm, dorsum of hand	Triceps, wrist extensors
Ulnar (C7-T1)	Anterior/medial forearm, 4th and 5th fingers	Ulnar flexion, flexor digitorum profundus for last two digits
Median (C6-T1)	Anterior/lateral forearm, palmer thumb, 1st, 2nd finger, half of 3rd finger	Thenar eminence, pronators

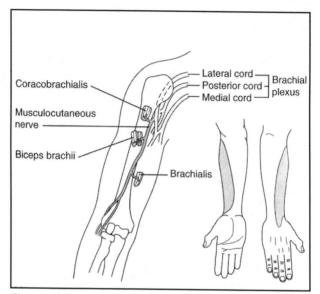

Figure 1. Motor and sensory distribution of musculocutaneous nerves (reprinted with permission from Magee D. *Orthopedic Physical Assessment*. 3rd ed. Philadelphia, Pa: WB Saunders; 1997).

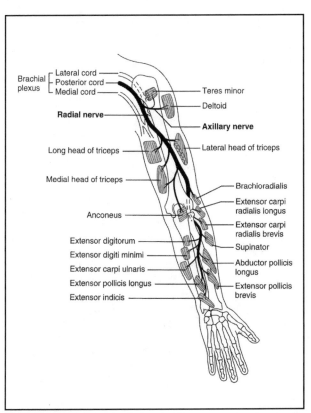

Figure 2. Distribution of radial and axillary nerves (reprinted with permission from Magee D. *Orthopedic Physical Assessment.* 3rd ed. Philadelphia, Pa: WB Saunders; 1997).

APPENDIX 12

Peripheral Nerve Innervations—Lower Extremity

Peripheral Nerve	Sensory Area	Manual Muscle Test (See Figures 1 through 5 for complete list)
Femoral	Medial thigh and leg	Quadriceps
Sciatic	Posterior thigh and leg	Hamstrings
Obturator	Mid anterior thigh	Adductors
Common peroneal	See deep and superficial peroneal	See deep and superficial peroneal
Deep peroneal	Web space between 1st and 2nd toes	Dorsiflexors
Superficial peroneal	Medial dorsal surface of foot	Evertors
Tibial	Posterior leg	Plantar flexors

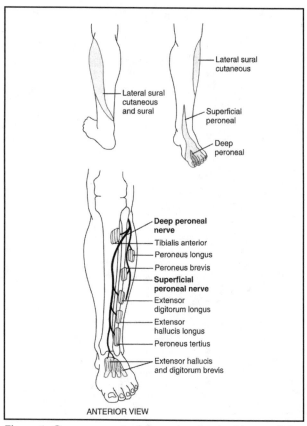

Figure 1. Common peroneal nerve (reprinted with permission from Magee D. *Orthopedic Physical Assessment.* 3rd ed. Philadelphia, Pa: WB Saunders; 1997).

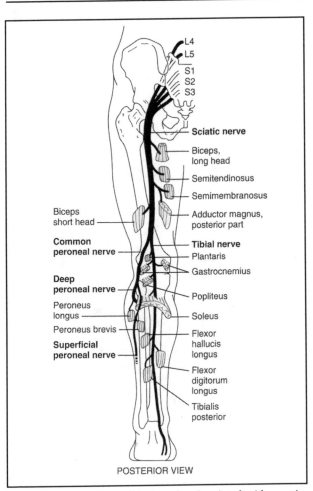

Figure 2. Sciatic nerve and its branches (reprinted with permission from Magee D. *Orthopedic Physical Assessment.* 3rd ed. Philadelphia, Pa: WB Saunders; 1997).

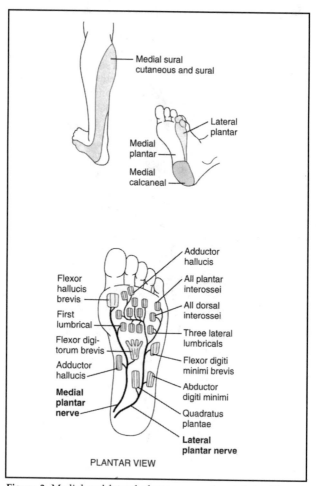

Figure 3. Medial and lateral plantar nerves (reprinted with permission from Magee D. *Orthopedic Physical Assessment*. 3rd ed. Philadelphia, Pa: WB Saunders; 1997).

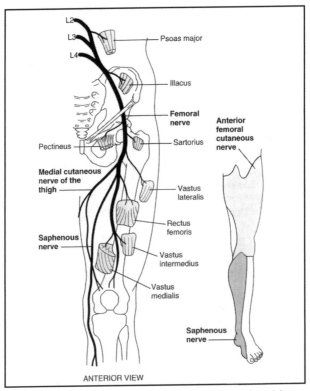

Figure 4. Femoral nerve (reprinted with permission from Magee D. *Orthopedic Physical Assessment.* 3rd ed. Philadelphia, Pa: WB Saunders; 1997).

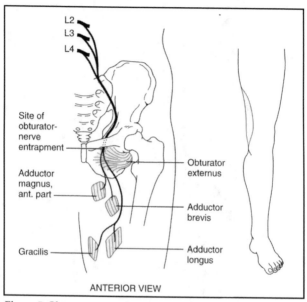

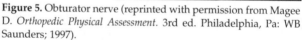

ANTERIOR VIEW

Figure 5. Obturator nerve (reprinted with permission from Magee D. *Orthopedic Physical Assessment.* 3rd ed. Philadelphia, Pa: WB Saunders; 1997).

APPENDIX 13

Muscle Grading

Manual Muscle Test (MMT) Grading

0	Absent	No contractions
1	Trace	Contraction felt, but unable to produce movement
2	Poor	Full ROM is possible with gravity removed
3	Fair	Partial ROM against gravity
4	Good	Resists moderate pressure
5	Normal	Resists maximal pressure—examiner cannot break resistance

APPENDIX 14

Grades of Pain

Grade

I   Patient complains of pain upon palpation

II   Patient complains of pain and winces upon palpation

III   Patient winces and withdraws the injured part upon palpation

IV   Patient will not allow palpation

APPENDIX 15

End Feel

Normal End Feel

Soft:	Created by soft tissue approximation (eg, elbow or knee flexion)
Firm:	Created by tissue stretch; stretch may be muscle/tendon, ligament, or capsule (eg, active or passive straight leg raise-hamstring tension)
Hard:	Bone on bone (eg, during elbow extension, the olecranon comes into contact with the olecranon fossa)

Abnormal End Feel

Soft:	Occurs sooner or later than normal or in a joint that normally has a firm or hard end feel
Firm:	Occurs sooner or later than normal or in a joint that normally has a soft or hard end feel
Hard:	Occurs sooner or later than normal or in a joint that normally has a firm or soft end feel (feels like a bony block or capsular tightness)
Springy block:	Hard end feel with slight spring, occurs sooner than normal end range
Empty:	Has no real end feel or pain inhibits reaching end ROM

Causes of Abnormal End Feels

Soft:	Inflammation (edema)
Firm:	Muscle spasm or shortening, capsular shortening
Hard:	Fracture, loose bodies, chondromalacia, myositis ossificans
Springy block:	Meniscal lesion
Empty:	Fracture, bursitis, abscess, acute joint inflammation, psychogenic origin

APPENDIX 16

Special Tests

Shoulder—Ligamentous Tests

Anterior Apprehension Test

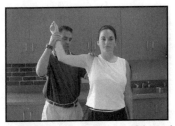

Patient is positioned with shoulder abducted (90 degrees), externally rotated, and elbow flexed (90 degrees). Examiner slowly applies external rotation force. Apprehension, pain, feeling of instability are positive signs.

Structure/condition tested: Anterior capsule

Jobe's Relocation Test (Fowler's sign)

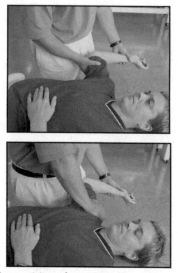

Patient is positioned supine. Examiner performs an anterior apprehension test followed by the same test with stabilization in a posterior direction. A positive sign is indicated by a reduction in pain.

Structure/condition tested: Anterior capsule

Posterior Apprehension Test

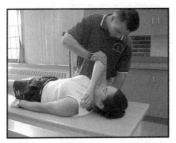

Patient is positioned supine with elbow flexed, shoulder flexed, and internally rotated. Examiner applies a posterior force. Apprehension, pain, or a feeling of instability are positive signs.

Structure/condition tested: Posterior capsule

Inferior Apprehension Test

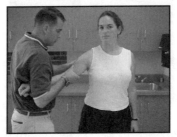

Patient is positioned with shoulder abducted. Examiner applies a downward traction. Apprehension, pain, sulcus, or a feeling of instability are positive signs.

Structure/condition tested: Inferior instability

Sulcus Sign

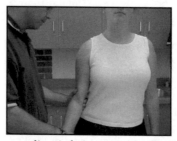

Examiner applies inferior traction to the humerus. Apprehension, pain, a sulcus, or widening of the space are positive signs.

Structure/condition tested: Inferior instability

AC Shear (AC Compression) Test

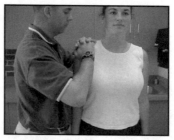

Examiner cups hands over the anterior and posterior joint and applies compression. Pain or movement of the clavicle are positive signs.

Structure/condition tested: AC ligament

O'Brien Test

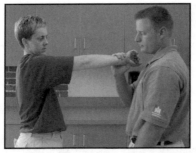

Patient is positioned with shoulder at 90 degrees flexion and internally rotated. Examiner applies internal rotation. Pain and/or audible "pop" are positive signs.

Structure/condition tested: Slap lesion

Clancy Test

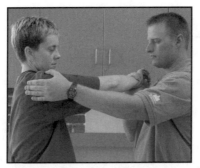

Test is similar to O'Brien except examiner applies a posterior force to the shoulder joint. Pain and/or palpable instability are positive signs.

Structure/condition tested: Slap lesion

Speeds Test

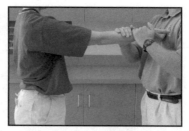

Patient is positioned standing or seated with shoulder flexed to 90 degrees, elbow extended, and forearm supinated. Examiner applies a downward (extension) pressure while patient resists with the extended elbow. Pain and weakness in the anterior shoulder indicate biceps tendonitis or tendon subluxation.

Structure/condition tested: Biceps tendonitis or subluxation

Yergason's Test

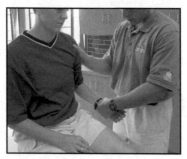

Patient is positioned standing or seated with elbow flexed and forearm supinated. The examiner palpates the bicipital groove and applies an elbow extension force along with shoulder external rotation and pronation to the forearm. The patient resists these motions. Pain or an audible "pop" indicate bicep subluxation.

Structure/condition tested: Biceps subluxation

Empty Can Test

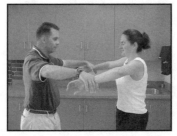

Patient is positioned in shoulder abduction, internal rotation, and slight horizontal flexion. Patient resists examiner's downward force. Pain or weakness are positive signs.

Structure/condition tested: Rotator cuff

Drop Arm Test

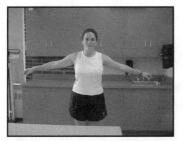

Patient is positioned in shoulder abduction; have the patient slowly lower the arms. The inability to control a slow movement is a positive sign.

Structure/condition tested: Rotator cuff-supraspinatus

Allen's Test

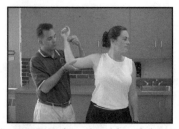

Patient is positioned in shoulder abduction and external rotation with the elbow flexed to 90 degrees. Have the patient rotate the neck to the opposite side. Check pulse. Absence or diminished pulse or radiating pain are positive signs.

Structure/condition tested: Thoracic outlet syndrome (TOS)

Adsons Maneuver

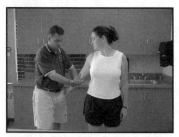

Patient is positioned in shoulder extension, external rotation, and neck extension and rotation to the same side. Check pulse. Absence or diminished pulse or radiating pain are positive signs.

Structure/condition tested: Thoracic outlet syndrome (TOS)

Halstead Maneuver

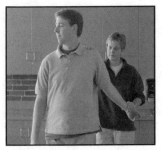

Patient is positioned in shoulder extension, external rotation, neck extension, and rotation to the opposite side. Examiner applies a downward traction force to the extremity. Absence or diminished pulse or radiating pain are positive signs.

Structure/condition tested: Thoracic outlet syndrome (TOS)

Costoclavicular Test

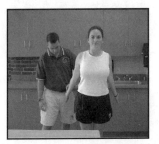

Patient maintains a military posture (shoulders retracted). The examiner applies extension and external rotation of the shoulder while checking the pulse. Absence or diminished pulse or radiating pain are positive signs.

Structure/condition tested: Thoracic outlet syndrome (TOS)

Roo's Test

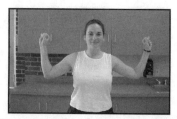

Patient is positioned in active abduction, external rotation. Patient opens and closes the fist for 3 minutes. Unable to complete the test, absence or diminished pulse, or radiating pain are positive signs.

Structure/condition tested: Thoracic outlet syndrome (TOS)

Cross-Over Impingement Test

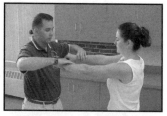

Patient is positioned in shoulder flexion (90 degrees). Examiner resists the patient's shoulder horizontal flexion. Pain and weakness are positive signs.

Structure/condition tested: Impingement. Anterior pain—biceps tendon, supraspinatus, or subscapularis impingement. Posterior pain—teres minor, infraspinatus, or capsular pathology.

Hawkins-Kennedy Impingement Sign

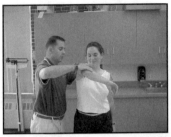

The patient's shoulder is flexed to 90 degrees. The examiner forcibly internally rotates the shoulder with elbow flexed to 90 degrees.

Structure/condition tested: Biceps tendon or supraspinatus impingement

Neer Impingement Sign

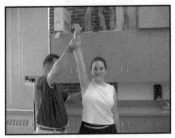

Examiner forcibly flexes the shoulder with shoulder internal rotation, elbow extended.

Structure/condition tested: Biceps tendon or supraspinatus impingement

Elbow—Ligamentous Tests

Valgus/Varus Stress Test

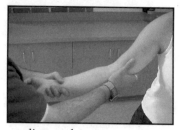

Examiner applies a valgus or varus stress to the joint.
Structure/condition tested: Collateral ligaments

Cozen's Test

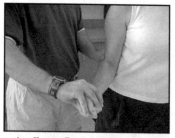

With patient's elbow flexed, examiner palpates the lateral epicondyle and resists the patient's wrist extension/radial deviation. Pain and weakness are positive signs.

Structure/condition tested: Lateral epicondylitis (extensors)

Mills' Test

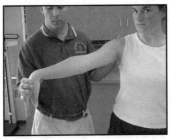

With the patient's elbow extended and pronated, apply passive wrist flexion. Pain at the epicondyle is a positive sign.

Structure/condition tested: Lateral epicondylitis (extensors)

Medial Epicondylitis Test

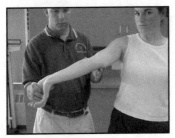

Same as above but the examiner apples passive wrist extension with the forearm in supination. Pain at the epicondyle is a positive sign.

Structure/condition tested: Medial epicondylitis (flexors)

Elbow Flexion Test

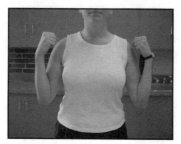

Patient is positioned in elbow flexion and asked to hold the position for 1 minute. Pain or numbness/tingling in the ulnar nerve distribution are positive signs.

Structure/condition tested: Ulnar nerve entrapment

Whartenberg's Sign

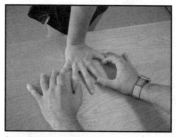

Patient's hand is positioned lying on a table. Examiner passively abducts the patient's fingers. Patient's inability to return 5th finger to the hand is a positive sign.

Structure/condition tested: Ulnar nerve neuropathy

Pronator Teres Syndrome

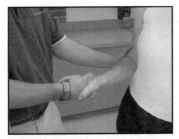

Examiner resists patient's pronation. Pain and/or numbness/tingling in median nerve distribution are positive signs.

Structure/condition tested: Median nerve entrapment

Tinel's Sign

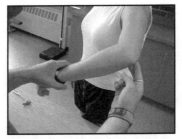

Examiner taps over the patient's ulnar nerve.
Structure/condition tested: Ulnar nerve injury

Hand/Wrist—Ligamentous Tests

Valgus/Varus Stress Test

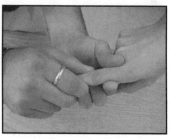

Examiner supports the proximal segment near the joint and applies a valgus/varus force.

Structure/condition tested: Interphalangeal joint collageral ligament

Phalen's Test

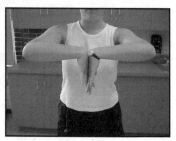

Patient places the dorsal surface of the hands together and pushes wrists into flexion. This position is held for 1 minute. Pain and/or paresthesia are positive signs.

Structure/condition tested: Carpal tunnel syndrome

Murphy's Sign

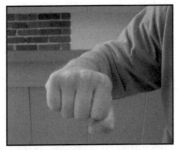

Patient is asked to make a fist. A positive test is indicated if the head of the 3rd metacarpal is level with the heads of the 2nd and 4th metacarpals.

Structure/condition tested: Lunate dislocation

Watson's Test (Scaphoid Shift Test)

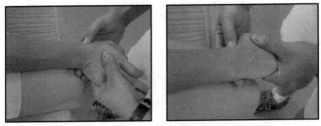

The patient is positioned seated with the arm pronated and resting on the thigh. The examiner stabilizes the distal end of the scaphoid and passively moves the wrist into full ulnar deviation and slight extension. The examiner then passively moves the joint into radial deviation and slight flexion. A positive test is indicated by a subluxation of the scaphoid dorsally above the rim of the radius and the patient complains of pain.

Structure/condition tested: Scaphoid/lunate instability

Tinel's Sign

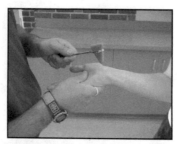

Examiner taps over the median or ulnar nerve as it crosses the dorsal surface of the wrist. Pain and/or paresthesia are positive signs.

Structure/condition tested: Median/ulnar nerve

Finkelstein's Test

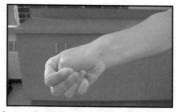

Patient places the thumb inside the closed fist and performs wrist ulnar deviation. Pain is a positive sign.

Structure/condition tested: de Quervain's disease

Thumb Hyperextension Test

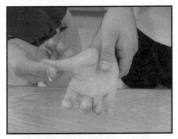

Examiner applies hyperextension force to the metacarpophalangeal (MCP) joint to assess ligamentous integrity.

Structure/condition tested: Volar plate

Bunnel/Littler Test

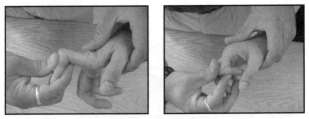

Assess flexion ROM of the PIP with the MCP slightly extended. Compare to ROM when MCP is slightly flexed.

Structure/condition tested: PIP contracture. Findings: Limited range with MCP extended, which indicates tight intrinsics; limited range with MCP flexed, which indicates capsular tightness.

Neck—Ligamentous Tests

Compression Test

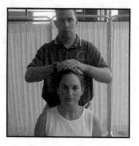

Patient is seated with head in neutral position. Examiner applies compression/axial load. Neck pain and especially radicular pain are positive signs.

Structure/condition tested: Nerve root compression

Foraminal Compression Test (Spurling's Test)

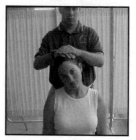

Patient is seated with neck laterally flexed to one side. Examiner applies compression/axial load. Neck pain and especially radicular pain are positive signs.

Structure/condition tested: Nerve root compression, foraminal compression

Jackson Compression Test

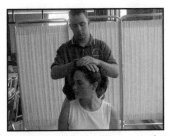

Patient is seated with neck rotated to one side. Examiner applies compression/axial load. Neck pain and especially radicular pain are positive signs.

Structure/condition tested: Nerve root compression

Maximum Cervical Compression Test

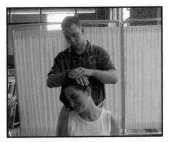

Patient is seated with neck laterally flexed and rotated to one side. Examiner applies compression/axial load. Neck pain and especially radicular pain are positive signs.

Structure/condition tested: Nerve root compression

Distraction Test

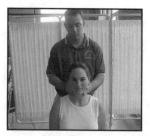

Patient is seated with neck in neutral position. Examiner applies distraction to the head/neck. The relief of symptoms is a positive sign.

Structure/condition tested: Nerve root compression

Shoulder Depression Test

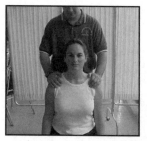

Patient is seated with neck laterally flexed to one side. Examiner depresses patient's opposite shoulder. Neck pain and especially radicular pain are positive signs.

Structure/condition tested: Brachial plexus traction injury and positive pain/radiculopathy along dermatome

Spine—Ligamentous Tests

Lasegues

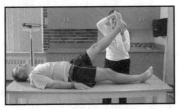

Examiner performs a passive straight leg raise (SLR) to the point of patient's pain. Examiner then lowers the leg until the patient's pain is gone. Patient is then asked to perform active dorsiflexion of the ankle.

Structure/condition tested: Nerve root involvement

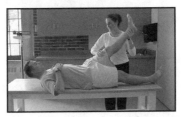

An alternate method is to have the patient perform active neck flexion. Back pain and especially radicular pain are positive signs.

Structure/condition tested: Nerve root involvement

Well Straight Leg Raise (SLR) Test

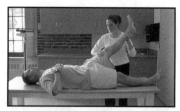

Examiner performs a passive SLR of the uninvolved limb. Back pain and especially radicular pain of the involved limb are positive signs.

Structure/condition tested: Nerve root involvement

Kernig (Brudzinski) Sign

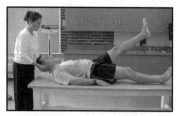

Similar to Lasegues, except patient performs active SLR of involved limb. Examiner provides passive neck flexion for the patient. Back pain and especially radicular pain are positive signs.

Structure/condition tested: Nerve root involvement

Milgrams Test

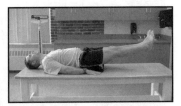

Patient performs a bilateral SLR and holds this position for 30 seconds. The inability to perform the test or the production of pain are positive signs.

Structure/condition tested: Nerve root involvement

Valsalva's Maneuver

Patient is asked to bear down (alternate method is to have patient blow into closed fist). Back pain and especially radicular pain are positive signs.

Structure/condition tested: Nerve root involvement

Bowstring Test (Cram/Popliteal Pressure Test)

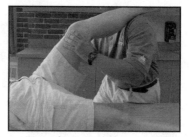

Patient is positioned supine. The examiner performs a passive SLR to the point of pain and then allows knee flexion until pain is relieved. The examiner then applies pressure to the popliteal space. A positive sign of pain indicates sciatic nerve compression or tension.

Structure/condition tested: Nerve root involvement

Facet Joint Test

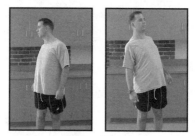

Patient extends, laterally flexes, and rotates trunk to same side. Pain is a positive sign.

Hoover Test (Malingering Test)

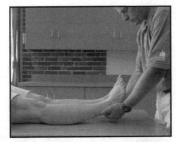

The patient is positioned supine. The examiner places one hand under each calcaneus between the patient and the table. The patient is asked to perform a straight leg raise. If the patient cannot raise the leg and the examiner does not feel pressure under the patient's heel, the patient may be malingering.

Structure/condition tested: Malingering

Sacroiliac Joint

FABER (Patrick's Test) Test

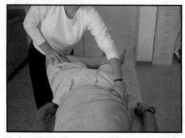

Flexion, ABduction, External Rotation. Patient is positioned supine with one ankle crossed over the opposite knee. Examiner applies pressure to the ASIS and knee of the crossed leg. The inability to move the thigh parallel to the table or the production of sacroiliac pain are positive signs.

Structure/condition tested: Sacroiliac dysfunction, hip internal rotation contracture

Yeoman's Test

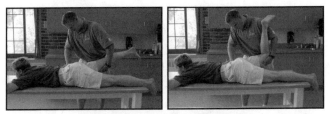

Patient is positioned prone. Examiner passively extends the hip first with the knee extended and then with knee flexed. Pain in the low back indicates lumbar involvement; pain in the sacroiliac area indicates anterior sacroiliac ligament injury, femoral nerve stretch; and pain in the anterior hip/thigh area indicates femoral nerve stretch.

Structure/condition tested: Sacroiliac dysfunction, lumbar involvement, femoral nerve stretch

Gapping Test

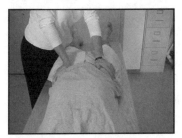

Patient is positioned supine. Examiner applies a "down and out" pressure to the iliac crests.

Structure/condition tested: Sacroiliac dysfunction

Squish Test

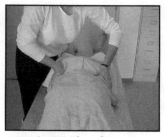

Same as the gapping test but the examiner applies pressure "down and in." Pain in the sacroiliac joint or radicular pain are positive signs.

Structure/condition tested: Sacroiliac dysfunction

Sacral Apex Test

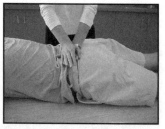

Patient is positioned prone. Examiner applies force straight down on the sacrum. Pain in the sacroiliac joint or radicular pain are positive signs.

Structure/condition tested: Sacroiliac dysfunction

Gaenslin's Test

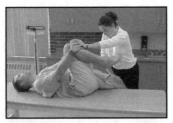

Patient is positioned supine near the edge of the examination table. The patient's limb is positioned over the edge of the table so as to allow passive hip extension and knee flexion. The opposite knee and hip are flexed and pressure is applied to both limbs. Pain in the sacroiliac joint or radicular pain are positive signs.

Structure/condition tested: Sacroiliac dysfunction

Hip—Ligamentous Tests

Sign of the Buttocks

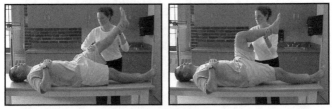

Examiner performs a passive SLR to the point of pain or the early end of range of motion. Examiner then attempts further hip flexion with knee flexed. No increase in hip flexion ROM is a positive sign for bursitis, tumor, or other hip joint pathology.

Structures/condition tested: Trochanteric bursistis, tumor

Ely's Test

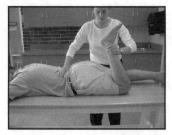

Patient is positioned prone with the knee flexed. The examiner applies further knee flexion. If the hip stays flat on table, this indicates normal flexibility (length) of the rectus femoris muscle.

Structure/condition tested: Rectus femoris contracture

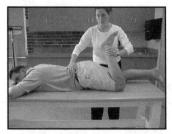

Hip flexion, causing the hip to raise off the table, is a positive sign indicating a tight rectus femoris.

Kendall Test

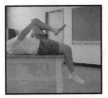

Patient is positioned supine near the end of the table with hip extended, knee flexed, and leg hanging off the edge of the table. Hip and knee flexion of the contralateral limb that causes the knee of the test leg to extend is a positive sign of rectus femoris contracture. Negative—knee stays flexed indicating normal flexibility (length) of the rectus femoris muscle.

Structure/condition tested: Rectus femoris contracture

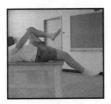

Positive Sign—knee extends, indicating a tight rectus femoris.

Thomas Test

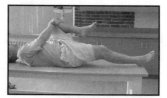

Similar to Kendall Test except the patient is positioned supine with the hip and knee extended. Hip and knee flexion of the contralateral limb that causes the hip and knee of the test leg to flex is a positive sign of hip flexor contracture (not rectus femoris). Negative—Hip and knee stay extended as the pelvis is tilted anteriorly. Positive—Hip flexes as the pelvis is "tilted" anteriorly, indicating tight hip flexors.

Structure/condition tested: Hip flexor contracture

Trendelenburg's Test

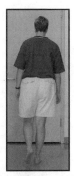

Examiner is positioned behind the patient. Patient is asked to stand on affected limb. If patient is unable to maintain a level pelvis, test is positive for weak gluteus medius.

Structure/condition tested: Gluteus medius weakness

Ober's Test

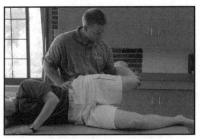

Patient is positioned side lying with the unaffected limb down. Examiner abducts and extends the hip with the knee in flexion. The examiner then passively lowers the hip into adduction. If adduction ROM is limited, the test is positive for tensor fascia contracture.

Structure/condition tested: Tensor fascia contracture

Knee—Ligamentous Tests

Anterior Draw Sign

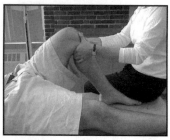

Patient is positioned supine with knee flexed to 90 degrees. Examiner grasps the tibia just distal to the knee joint and applies an anterior force, assessing the integrity of the anterior cruciate ligament.

Structure/condition tested: Anteromedial bundle of the anterior cruciate ligament

Slocum

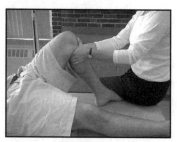

A variation on the anterior draw sign in which the tibia is rotated internally and externally prior to the application of the anterior draw.

Structure/condition tested: anterior cruciate ligament

Lachman's Test

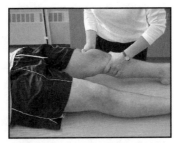

Patient is positioned supine. Examiner grasps the patient's leg just above and below the knee and positions the knee in slight flexion (approximately 10 to 15 degrees). While stabilizing the thigh, the examiner applies an anterior force to the tibia.

Structure/condition tested: Posterolateral bundle of the anterior cruciate ligament

Pivot Shift Test

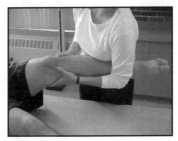

Patient is positioned supine. Examiner grasps the patient's leg just above and below the knee and positions the knee in slight flexion. The examiner applies a valgus force and internal tibial rotation while further flexing the knee. As the knee is flexed to approximately 30 to 40 degrees, the tibia will shift posteriorly back into position.

Structure/condition tested: anterior cruciate ligament

Posterior Draw Sign

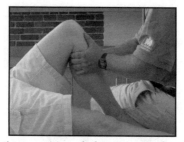

With patient positioned the same as for the anterior draw sign, the examiner applies a posterior force over the tibial tubercle to stress the posterior cruciate ligament.

Structure/condition tested: posterior cruciate ligament

Posterior Sag Test (Profile Test)

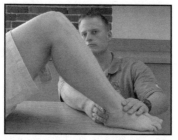

With the patient positioned the same as for the anterior/posterior draw sign, observe the tibial tubercle for a posterior sag in comparison to the opposite limb.

Structure/condition tested: posterior cruciate ligament

Godfrey's Test

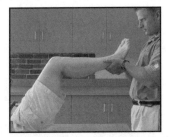

With the patient positioned supine with the hips and knees at 90 degrees, observe the tibial tubercle for a posterior sag in comparison to the opposite limb.

Structure/condition tested: posterior cruciate ligament

Valgus Stress

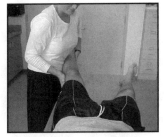

The patient is positioned supine. The examiner grasps the patient's lower leg and applies a valgus force at the knee to stress the medial collateral and capsular ligaments.

Structure/condition tested: medial collateral ligament/medial capsule

Varus Stress Test

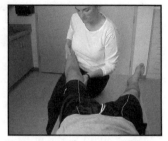

The patient is positioned supine. The examiner grasps the patient's lower leg and applies a varus force at the knee to stress the lateral collateral and capsular ligaments.

Structure/condition tested: lateral collateral ligament/lateral capsule

Knee—Meniscal Tests

Bounce Home Test

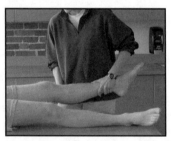

The patient is positioned supine with the knee slightly flexed. The examiner allows the knee to drop into extension. If ROM is limited or end range is springy, a meniscal lesion could be the cause.

Apley's Compression Test

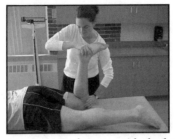

The patient is positioned prone with the knee flexed to 90 degrees. The examiner grasps the patient's foot and applies a longitudinal force along the shaft of the tibia and rotates the tibia internally and externally. Pain, locking, or catching are positive signs for meniscal tear.

Structure/condition tested: Meniscus

Apley's Distraction Test

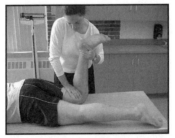

Positioning is the same as for Apley's compression test except that a distraction force is applied by grasping the patient's ankle and stabilizing the opposite thigh. A relief of pain indicates meniscal tear.

Structure/condition tested: Meniscus

McMurray Test

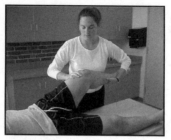

The patient is positioned supine. The examiner grasps the patient's leg just above and below the knee. The examiner applies a valgus and varus force combining internal and external tibial rotation while flexing and extending the knee. Pain, locking, or catching are positive signs for meniscal tear.

Structure/condition tested: Meniscus

Noble Compression Test

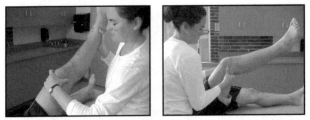

Patient is positioned supine. The examiner palpates the lateral femoral epicondyle while flexing and extending the patient's knee. Pain as the Iliotibial band crosses over the lateral epicondyle is a positive sign.

An alternate method is to have the patient perform active knee extension.

Structure/condition tested: Iliotibial band friction syndrome

Patella Apprehension Test

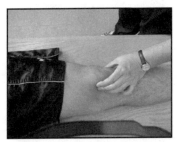

Patient is positioned supine. With knee extended and patient relaxed, the examiner applies a gentle lateral force to the patella. A patient who has subluxed the patella will be apprehensive (ie, will contract quads or pull away).

Structure/condition tested: Patella subluxation

Patella Tracking Test

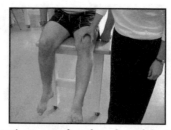

With the patient seated at the edge of the table, knee at 90 degrees, the examiner places the hand over the lateral edges of the patella. Have the patient slowly extend and flex the knee through full range of motion. Patella should move superiorly and slightly laterally in a smooth coordinated motion.

Structure/condition tested: Patella Tracking

Crunch/Grind Test

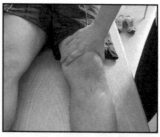

The patient is positioned supine with the knee extended and leg relaxed. The examiner applies a stabilizing force just proximal to the patella. The patient then *slowly* contracts the quadriceps. *Warning*—this test is painful even to asymptomatic individuals. Apply cautiously.

Structure/condition tested: Chondromalacia

Foot/Ankle—Ligamentous Tests

Anterior Draw Test

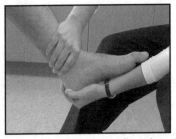

The patient is seated with knee flexed to 90 degrees. The examiner stabilizes the tibia with one hand and grasps the calcaneus and "draws" (pulls) forward to assess the integrity of the ligaments.

Structure/condition tested: Anterior talofibular, deltoid, anterior tibiofibular

Anterior Draw Test 2

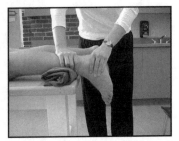

The patient is positioned prone with the foot hanging off the edge of the table, with padding under the distal tibia. The examiner applies a downward (anterior) pressure to the calcaneus to assess the integrity of the ligaments.

Structure/condition tested: Anterior talofibular, deltoid, anterior tibiofibular

Talar Tilt

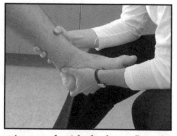

The patient is seated with the knee flexed to 90 degrees. The examiner stabilizes the tibia, grasps the calcaneus, and applies inversion and eversion stresses. It is performed in neutral, dorsiflexion, and plantar flexion.

Structure/condition tested: Inversion—neutral-calcaneofibular, dorsi-post talofibular, plantar-anterior talofibular. Eversion—deltoid

Kleiger Test

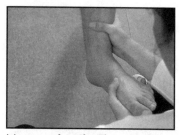

Same position as talar tilt. The examiner stabilizes the tibia, grasps the foot, and applies a lateral rotation force to stress the ligaments.

Structure/condition tested: Deltoid, anterior tibiofibular

Midtarsal Test

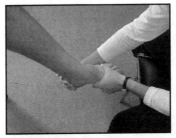

Same position as talar tilt. The examiner stabilizes the calcaneus, grasps the midfoot (approximately over the first metatarsophalangeal joint), and applies a torsion (twisting motion) to stress the midtarsal ligaments.

Structure/condition tested: Midtarsal ligaments

Thompson's Test

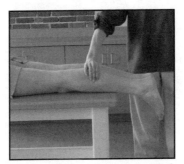

The patient is positioned prone with knee extended. The examiner grasps the triceps surae and squeezes. No plantar flexion is a sign of a ruptured Achilles' tendon.

Structure/condition tested: Achilles' tendon rupture

Bump/Tap Test

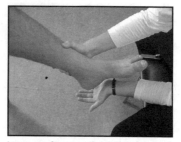

The examiner applies a vibratory force along the long axis of the lower leg by "bumping/tapping" the calcaneus.
Structure/condition tested: Fibular fracture

Toe Distract Test

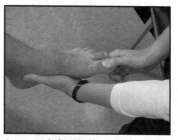

The examiner stabilizes the proximal segment and applies a traction force to the distal segment.
Structure/condition tested: Ligament sprain

Toe Tap Test

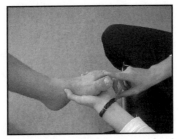

The examiner applies a light tap to the long axis of the toe.

Structure/condition tested: Fracture

APPENDIX 17

NATA Code of Ethics

(Reprinted with permission of NATA ©
NATA Code of Ethics; 1999)

Preamble

The Code of Ethics of the National Athletic Trainers' Association has been written to make the membership aware of the principles of ethical behavior that should be followed in the practice of athletic training. The primary goal of the Code is the assurance of high quality health care. The Code presents aspirational standards of behavior that all members should strive to achieve.

The principles cannot be expected to cover all specific situations that may be encountered by the practicing athletic trainer, but should be considered representative of the spirit with which athletic trainers should make decisions. The principles are written generally and the circumstances of a situation will determine the interpretation and application of a given principle and of the Code as a whole. Whenever there is a conflict between the Code and legality, the laws prevail. The guidelines set forth in this Code are subject to continual review and revision as the athletic training profession develops and changes.

PRINCIPLE 1:

Members shall respect the rights, welfare and dignity of all individuals.

1.1 Members shall not discriminate against any legally protected class.

1.2 Members shall be committed to providing competent care consistent with both the requirements and the limitations of their profession.

1.3 Members shall preserve the confidentiality of privileged information and shall not release such information to a third party not involved in the patient's care unless the person consents to such release or release is permitted or required by law.

PRINCIPLE 2:
Members shall comply with the laws and regulations governing the practice of athletic training.

2.1 Members shall comply with applicable local, state, and federal laws and institutional guidelines.

2.2 Members shall be familiar with and adhere to all National Athletic Trainers' Association guidelines and ethical standards.

2.3 Members are encouraged to report illegal or unethical practice pertaining to athletic training to the appropriate person or authority.

2.4 Members shall avoid substance abuse and, when necessary, seek rehabilitation for chemical dependency.

PRINCIPLE 3:
Members shall accept responsibility for the exercise of sound judgment.

3.1 Members shall not misrepresent in any manner, either directly or indirectly, their skills, training, professional credentials, identity, or services.

3.2 Members shall provide only those services for which they are qualified via education and/or experience and by pertinent legal regulatory process.

3.3 Members shall provide services, make referrals, and seek compensation only for those services that are necessary.

PRINCIPLE 4:
Members shall maintain and promote high standards in the provision of services.

4.1 Members shall recognize the need for continuing education and participate in various types of educational activities that enhance their skills and knowledge.

4.2 Members who have the responsibility for employing and evaluating the performance of other staff members shall fulfill such responsibility in a fair, considerate, and equitable manner, on the basis of clearly enunciated criteria.

4.3 Members who have the responsibility for evaluating the performance of employees, supervisors, or students, are encouraged to share evaluations with them and allow them the opportunity to respond to those evaluations.

4.4 Members shall educate those whom they supervise in the practice of athletic training with regard to the Code of Ethics and encourage their adherence to it.

4.5 Whenever possible, members are encouraged to participate and support others in the conduct and communication of research and educational activities that may contribute knowledge for improved patient care, patient or student education, and the growth of athletic training as a profession.

4.6 When members are researchers or educators, they are responsible for maintaining and promoting ethical conduct in research and educational activities.

PRINCIPLE 5:
Members shall not engage in any form of conduct that constitutes a conflict of interest or that adversely reflects on the profession.

5.1 The private conduct of the member is a personal matter to the same degree as is any other person's except when such conduct compromises the fulfillment of professional responsibilities.

5.2 Members of the National Athletic Trainers' Association and others serving on the Association's committees or acting as consultants shall not use, directly or by implication, the Association's name or logo or their affiliation with the Association in the endorsement of products or services.

5.3 Members shall not place financial gain above the welfare of the patient being treated and shall not participate in any arrangement that exploits the patient.

5.4 Members may seek remuneration for their services that is commensurate with their services and in compliance with applicable law.

Reporting of Ethics Violations

Anyone having information regarding allegations of ethical violations, and wishing to supply such information to NATA, shall supply this information, with as much specificity and documentation as possible, to NATA's Executive Director or Chair of the Ethics Committee.

Information need not be supplied in writing, and the reporting individual need not identify him or herself. Information, however, that is too vague, cannot be substantiated without the assistance of the reporting person, or information where, in the opinion of the NATA Executive Director or Ethics Chair, there is no need for anonymity for the reporting individual will not be forwarded for action by the committee.

An individual may report information on the condition that the individual's name or certain other facts be kept confidential. NATA may proceed with an investigation subject to such a condition; however, NATA must inform the reporting individual that at some point in the investigation.

NATA may determine that it cannot proceed further without disclosing some of the confidential information, either to the applicant or member under investigation or to some other party. A reporting individual, upon receiving this information from NATA, may decide whether or not to allow the information to be revealed. If the reporting individual decides that the necessary information must remain confidential, NATA may be required to close the unfinished investigation for lack of necessary information. Individuals are strongly encouraged to provide relevant information, with as much detail as possible, in writing to:

NATA
Ethics Investigations
2952 Stemmons Frwy
Dallas, TX 75247-6196

as of 12/17/1999

APPENDIX 18

NATA Membership Policies and Privileges

(Reprinted with permission of NATA © *NATA Membership—
Policies and Privileges*; 1999)

Membership Categories

Individuals may apply for NATA membership in one of the below categories. Each category description outlines the requirements for membership in the category and the voting privileges, if any, for that category. Individuals who apply for membership in a category for which they are not eligible will be automatically transferred by NATA to the appropriate category.

CERTIFIED

This membership category is open only to individuals possessing current NATABOC certification. Certified membership has four subcategories: regular, graduate student, international and retired. Certified regular and graduate student members may vote on association matters and may hold office within NATA. Only certified individuals enrolled as full-time graduate students in an accredited college or university may select the graduate student subcategory. Certified student members pay the student membership fee. Certified individuals living overseas in an area not included in any current District are certified international members. Certified international members may choose a District and pay dues for that affiliation, if they wish to do so and the District policy allows it.

ASSOCIATE

This membership category is open to individuals who are working professionally in athletics, education, research, medicine, or an allied health or other profession related to athletic training. Associate members may not vote or hold office within NATA.

STUDENT

This membership category is open only to individuals meeting one of the below criteria. Members in this category may not vote or hold office within NATA.

A. Non-certified individuals enrolled as full-time graduate students in an accredited college or university; or,

B. Individuals currently making progress toward the fulfillment of the requirements for NATABOC certification by participating in an internship or approved curriculum program under the supervision of an NATA certified athletic trainer.

INTERNATIONAL

This membership category is open only to non-certified individuals who do not have a permanent address in the United States or Canada. Members of this category are not eligible for district affiliation and may not vote or hold office in NATA. Individuals who are stationed temporarily overseas with the military are not eligible for membership in this category.

SUPPLIER

This membership category is open only to corporations which are suppliers and/or manufacturers of athletic training materials, supplies, equipment or services. Each supplier member will be entitled to designate one individual as the corporation's representative to NATA.

Members of this category are not eligible for district affiliation and may not vote or hold office, within NATA. Supplier members will be entitled to member discounts rates on a variety of products and services, including reduced advertising rates in NATA's publications and reduced exhibit booth rental fees at the Annual Meeting.

NATA Membership Policies

The membership year is January 1 through December 31. Annual membership fee renewal invoices are mailed each year on November 1 and are due no later than January 1. After February 15, individuals who have not renewed their membership are placed on suspension. Suspended individuals who do not renew their membership by September 30 are removed from the NATA membership records.

Individuals who let their membership lapse and then rejoin NATA will be charged a $25.00 application processing fee ($15.00 for student applicants). This fee is non-refundable.

The annual membership fee consists of a national fee and a district fee (with the exception of supplier members, who do not have district affiliation). Both fees must be paid in full each year. The annual membership fees are listed on the back of the application form and must be submitted with the membership application. The National membership fee is prorated every four months for new members. If a membership application is denied, the annual membership fee will be returned to the applicant.

Members will be assigned to the district that corresponds with the mailing address maintained for them by NATA. Students are required to use their permanent home address for their NATA membership. All others are requested to use their work address.

The National Athletic Trainer's Association (NATA)

We hope that by now you have read our information about how membership in the National Athletic Trainers' Association (NATA) can benefit you and have decided to join.

Before completing the membership application, we encourage you to familiarize yourself with the NATA membership policies and categories described here. If you have any questions that this website does not answer, please feel free to contact our membership department at the following:

NATA
2952 Stemmons Freeway
Dallas, TX 75247-6103
214-637-6282
FAX 214-637-2206

We look forward to receiving your membership application and to including you as an NATA member.

APPENDIX 19

NATABOC Standards of Professional Practice

(Reprinted with permission of NATABOC ©
Standards and Disciplinary; 2000)

Preamble

The Professional Practice and Disciplinary Process of the NATABOC is intended to assist and inform the public, certificate holders, and candidates for certification, of the NATABOC Standards of Professional Practice and the Disciplinary Process relative to professional conduct and disciplinary procedures.

The NATABOC conducts a certification program for athletic trainers and has established a recertification requirement for certified athletic trainers (ATC). The NATABOC affirms that, after a candidate has successfully passed the certification examination, the Standards of Professional Practice for entry into the profession of athletic training have been satisfied.

The NATABOC does not express an opinion on the competence or warrant job performance of certificants; however, it is expected that a certificant or candidate of certification agrees to comply at all times to the following Standards of Professional Practice.

Standards of Professional Practice

A. Standards of Professional Practice for Athletic Training—Direct Service: The following are minimal standards. Each one is essential for the practice of athletic training.

Standard 1: Direction

The athletic trainer renders service or treatment under the direction of a physician or dentist.

Standard 2: Injury and On-Going Care Services

All services should be documented in writing by the athletic trainer and shall become part of the athlete's permanent records.

Standard 3: Documentation

The athletic trainer shall accept responsibility for recording details of the athlete's health status.

Documentation shall include:

1. Athlete's name and any other identifying information
2. Referral source (doctor, dentist)
3. Date; initial assessment, results and database
4. Program plan and estimated length
5. Program methods, results and revisions
6. Date of discontinuation and summary
7. Athletic trainer's signature.

Standard 4: Confidentiality

The athletic trainer shall maintain confidentiality as determined by law and shall accept responsibility for communication assessment results, program plans, and progress with other persons involved in the athlete's program.

Standard 5: Initial Assessment

Prior to treatment, the athletic trainer shall assess the athlete's level of functioning. The athlete's input shall be considered an integral part of the initial assessment.

Standard 6: Program Planning

The athletic training program objectives shall include long- and short-term goals and an appraisal of those which the athlete can realistically be expected to achieve from the program. Assessment measures to determine effectiveness of the program shall be incorporated into the plan.

Standard 7: Program Discontinuation

The athletic trainer, with collaboration of the physician or dentist, shall recommend discontinuation of the athletic training service when the athlete has received optimal benefit of the program. The athletic trainer, at the time of discontinuation, shall note the final assessment of the athlete's status.

B. Standards of Professional Practice for Athletic Training—Service Programs

Standard 1: Objectives

Basic to the development of any program are its intended purposes. Objectives and applicable policies should be clearly outlined for each activity, such as: athletic treatment, education of personnel, supervision and interdisciplinary relations. The objectives of the service program should implement those of the institution itself.

Standard 2: Planning

Each objective should be supported by detailed plans for its implementation.

Standard 3: Evaluation

Objective methods of data collection and analysis should be used in relation to each component of the program to determine the need for service, assess its effectiveness and indicate a need for change.

Standard 4: Types of Services Offered

Athletic training is appropriately a health service offered under the direction of a physician or dentist for the prevention, immediate care, management/disposition and reconditioning of athletic injuries.

Standard 5: Personnel

The service program should be directed by a National Athletic Trainers' Association Board of Certification, Inc (NATABOC) Certified Athletic Trainer who has met the qualifications established by the NATABOC. Education, qualifications and experience of all other personnel should meet existing standards and should be appropriate to their duties.

Standard 6: Facilities and Budget

Space, equipment, supplies and a continuing budget should be provided by the institution and should be adequate in amount, variety and quality to facilitate the implementation of the service program.

Standard 7: Records

Objective, permanent records of each aspect of the service program should (1) indicate date, name of physician or dentist referral; (2) initial evaluation and assessment; (3) treatment or services rendered, with date; (4) dates of subsequent follow-up care.

Standard 8: Reports

Written reports on each aspect of the service program should be made annually.

Disciplinary Process

A. Standards of Professional Practice—Revocation of Certification:

The NATABOC may revoke or otherwise take action with regard to the application or certification of an individual in the case of:

1. Ineligibility for certification

2. Irregularity in connection with any certification application or examination;

3. Unauthorized possession, use, access, or distribution of certification examinations, score-reports, answer sheets,

certificates, certificant or applicant files, documents, or other materials

4. Material misrepresentation or fraud in any statement to the NATABOC or to the public, including, but not limited to, statements made to assist the applicant, certificant, or another apply for, obtain, or retain certification

5. Gross or repeated negligence or malpractice in professional work, which includes releasing confidential medical information of athletes or others with whom the certificant or applicant has a professional relationship

6. The conviction of, plea of guilty, or plea of nolo contendere (no contest) to a felony or misdemeanor which is directly related to public health, athletic care, or education. This includes but is not limited to rape, sexual abuse of a child or athlete, actual or threatened use of a weapon of violence; the prohibited sale or distribution of controlled substance, or its possession with the intent of distribute, or use of position of the athletic trainer improperly to influence the outcome or score of an athletic contest or event or in connection with any gambling activity

7. Not adhering to the eligibility requirements for certification candidacy or recertification requirements and the Standards of Professional Practice of the Profession.

B. Disciplinary committee and Panels

1. The NATABOC, by a majority vote, shall appoint three persons who are certified athletic trainers to the Professional Practice and Discipline Committee. When necessary, the NATABOC, by a majority vote, shall appoint three persons who are certified athletic trainers (i) a Hearing Panel, and/or (ii) an Appeals Panel, to consider alleged violations of any Application or Certification Standard set forth in Section I C (1)-(7) after review and decision by the Professional Practice and Discipline Committee. These Panels may be established as standing Panels. The Hearing and Appeals Panels shall be composed of three full-voting members and up to four non-voting (substitute) members.

2. A quorum of either the Committee or a Panel consists of three full-voting members, and Committee and Panel action shall be determined by a majority vote. Committee and Panel members may serve in only one capacity at a time. Committee and Panel members may not consider any matter that came before them prior to their service on the Committee or Panel. Committee and Panel members may not serve in any situation where their impartiality or the presence of actual or apparent conflict of interest might reasonably be questioned.

3. When a vacancy of a full-voting member occurs in any of the panels as a result of resignation, unavailability, or disqualification, the Executive Director of the NATABOC shall designate a full-voting member from the substitute members.

C. Review Process

Whenever the Executive Director receives allegations, which raise an issue under A (1)-(7), Standards of Professional Practice of the Profession, the Executive Director shall transmit such allegations to the Chair of the Professional Practice and Discipline Committee. If the Committee determines that no good cause exists to question eligibility or compliance with the Standards of Professional Practice, no further action shall be taken. However, if the Committee determines by majority vote that good cause does exist, it shall direct the transmittal to the applicant or certificant by certified mail or tracked courier, return receipt requested, of a letter containing a statement of the factual allegations constituting the alleged violation and the disciplinary standard allegedly violated. The letter shall also include the following recitation of rights and procedures: (1) the applicant or certificant shall have fifteen days in which to respond to the allegations, provide comments regarding appropriate sanctions, and request an oral hearing if he or she disputes the allegations; (2) sanctions may be imposed if the allegations are determined to be true by the Committee or a Disciplinary Panel, or if the applicant or certificant fails to submit a timely response; (3) the applicant or certificant will be deemed to consent to the imposition of sanctions by the Committee if he or she does not dispute the truthfulness of the allegations; (4) the applicant or certificant must appear in person if he or she requests a hearing; (5) the applicant or certificant may be represented by counsel at the hearing, may present evidence on his or her own behalf, and may examine or cross-examine any witness under oath.

D. Hearing

If an applicant or certificant disputes the allegations and requests a hearing:

1. The Chair shall: (a) forward the allegations and response of the applicant or certificant to the Hearing Panel; (b) schedule a hearing before the Hearing Panel after the request is received; (c) send by certified mail or tracked courier, return receipt requested, a Notice of Hearing to the applicant or certificant. The Notice of Hearing shall include a statement of the time and place of the hearing as selected by the Executive Director after consultation with the Chair of the Hearing Panel.

2. The Hearing Panel shall maintain an audiotaped or written transcript of the proceedings.

3. The NATABOC and the applicant or certificant may make opening statements, present documents and testimony, examine and cross-examine witnesses under oath, make closing statements, and present written briefs as schedule by the Hearing Panel.

4. The Hearing Panel shall determine all matters relating to the hearing. The hearing and related matters shall be determined on the record by majority vote. Formal rules of evidence shall not apply. Relevant evidence may be admitted. Disputed questions shall be determined by majority vote of the Panel.

E. Appeal

The applicant or certificant may appeal to the Appeals Panel a decision by the Hearing Panel regarding the truthfulness of the allegations and may appeal a decision by either the Committee or the Hearing Panel regarding the imposition of sanctions. An appeal must be filed within thirty days of the applicant or certificant's receipt of the decision through the submission of a written appeals statement of the Executive Director of the NATABOC. The NATABOC may file a written response to the appeals statement of the applicant or certificant. The Appeals Panel shall render a decision on the record without oral hearing, although written briefing may be submitted.

F. Decision

The decisions of the Committee, Hearing, and Appeals Panels shall be rendered in writing. A decision by the Hearing or Appeals panels shall contain factual findings, conclusions of law, and any sanctions applied. It shall be transmitted to the applicant or certificant by certified mail or tracked courier, return receipt requested.

G. Sanctions

Sanctions for violation of any NATABOC Standard may include one ore more of the following:

1. Denial or suspension of eligibility
2. Revocation
3. Non-renewal
4. Censure
5. Reprimand
6. Suspension
7. Training or other corrective action
8. Delinquent status
9. Reports; and conditions relating to the above.

H. Emergency Procedure

Whenever the Committee determines that there is cause to believe that a threat of immediate and irreparable injury to the health of the public exists, the Committee shall forward the allegations to the Hearing Panel. The Hearing Panel shall hear the matter by immediate telephone or other expedited notice and hearing procedure. If the Hearing Panel determines that a threat of immediate and irreparable injury to the public exists, certification may be suspended for up to 60 days pending full hearing under the procedure described above.

I. Release of Information

The individual applicant or certificant authorizes the NATABOC and its agents to communicate any information relating to the NATABOC application and/or certification, to state and federal authorities, employers, other applicants and certificants, educational programs, and others by means of newsletter or otherwise.

J. Waiver and Release

The individual releases, discharges, and exonerates the NATABOC, its officers, directors, employees, committee members, agents, and any person furnishing documents, records, and other information relating to the individual's eligibility, certification, or recertification from any and all liability of any nature and kind, arising out of the furnishing or inspection of such documents, records, or other information, and any investigation, evaluation, and communication regarding the individual's eligibility, certification, or recertification, made by the NATABOC.

K. Submission of Information to the NATABOC

Persons concerned with possible violations of NATABOC Standards of Professional Practice shall identify the persons alleged to be involved and the facts concerning the alleged conduct in as much detail and specificity as possible with the available documentation, in a written statement addressed to the Executive Director of the NATABOC. The statement should include the name, address, and telephone number of the person making the statement and others who may have knowledge of facts concerning the alleged violation.

Requirements To Maintain Certification
I. Overview

The NATABOC has established that all certified athletic trainers must obtain a predetermined amount of continuing education units (CEUs) with a three-year reporting term. This predetermined amount of CEUs is prorated based on the individual's year of certification. Each individual is also required to submit proof of current CPR certification at least once during that three-year term. Newly certified athletic trainers will be advised, when they receive their certification notice, of their continuing education requirement, as well as other information about the NATABOC's continuing education requirement.

The NATABOC has established the following certified status categories: ACTIVE, INACTIVE, SUSPENDED, VOLUNTARILY RESIGNED, DELINQUENT, and REVOKED.

II. Certified Status Categories
A. Active Status Policies:
(The following applies to the 2000-2002 CEU term)

1. The minimum number of CEU's required by December 31, 2002, for certified athletic trainers who were certified by December 31, 1999 is 80 units; those certified during 2000 will be required to obtain 55 units; and those certified in 2000 to obtain 25 units. Continuing education (recertification) requirements for athletic trainers certified in 2002 will begin with the 2003-2005 continuing education term. The NATABOC will provide all individuals who satisfy their continuing education requirements with a certificate for public display.

2. CPR certification must be current at the time the CEU reporting sheet is submitted.

3. Individuals should refer to the 2000-2002 NATABOC Continuing Education File Folder for specific guidelines and directions.

4. Failure to satisfy the NATABOC continuing education requirements can result in SUSPENSION or REVOCATION of an individual's certification. The status of a certified athletic trainer who does not satisfy the continuing education requirements by the end of a continuing education term will be changed from ACTIVE to SUSPENDED. If, after six months of the date of suspension, the individual's continuing education requirement has not been met, his or her certification will be REVOKED.

5. The National Athletic Trainers' Association (NATA) reimburses the NATABOC for recording and processing continuing education records for its members who were certified by the NATABOC. Certified athletic trainers who are not NATA members will be assessed an annual certification fee. Non-payment of this fee can result in a sanction by the NATABOC. The status of an individual who does not pay the annual certification fee will be changed to DELINQUENT. An individual who is listed as DELINQUENT after February 1 of each year will be changed to the classification of SUSPENDED. If, by June 1 of each year, the appropriate fee has not been submitted to the NATABOC, the certified athletic trainer's certification will be REVOKED.

6. A certified athletic trainer who has had his or her certification REVOKED must complete the entire entry-level certification process (satisfy current requirements and pass the entry-level certification examination) in order to regain ACTIVE status.

B. Inactive Policies

1. A certified athletic trainer who wishes to have his or her certification status changed from ACTIVE to INACTIVE can request this through the NATABOC. Application must be made to the NATABOC. A nonrefundable fee must accompany the application each year.

2. Examples of those who might desire INACTIVE status are:

a) an individual on active military duty or in the Peace Corps

b) an individual not currently practicing in the field of athletic training

c) an individual suffering serious medical problems.

3. While classified as INACTIVE, the certified athletic trainer does not have to obtain continuing education units.

4. While classified as INACTIVE, the certified athletic trainer agrees not to do the following:

a) serve as a supervisor of students who are satisfying the athletic training requirements for certification eligibility

b) serve as a model or examiner for the NATABOC certification examination

c) represent him or herself to the public as a practicing certified athletic trainer or use the initials "ATC" or "C.A.T" after his or her name.

5. If during a continuing education term a certified athletic trainer requests to have his or her status changed from INACTIVE to ACTIVE, he or she will be advised of the number of prorated CEUs required during that term, including current CPR certification.

6. A certified athletic trainer whose status is classified as INACTIVE for three years must attain a passing score on the written simulation section of the NATABOC certification examination in order to maintain his or her certified status.

7. A certified athletic trainer who requests INACTIVE status for three years and fails to take and pass the simulation section of the NATABOC certification examination will have his or her status changed to SUSPENDED. If the certified athletic trainer does not pass the simulation section within one year of the date of SUSPENSION, his or her certification status will be revoked.

8. A certified athletic trainer who has had his or her certification REVOKED must complete the entire entry-level

certification process (satisfy current requirements and pass the entry-level certification examination) in order to regain ACTIVE status.

C. Suspended

1. A certified athletic trainer who fails to satisfy the NATABOC continuing education requirements will be suspended. While suspended the athletic trainer cannot:

a. serve as a supervisor of students who are satisfying athletic training requirements for certification eligibility;

b. serve as a model or examiner for the NATABOC certification examination; or

c. represent him or herself to the public as a practicing certified athletic trainer or use the initials "ATC" or "C.A.T" after his or her name.

2. Regulatory agencies, the public, or employers who request to verify the status of an athletic trainer are only told that an athletic trainer who is suspended is not in good standing.

3. The NATABOC annually sends lists of athletic trainers not in good standing to state regulatory agencies who recognize the NATABOC credential for state licensing/registration purposes.

D. Voluntary Resigned Status Policies

1. A certified athletic trainer who wishes to voluntarily resign his or her certified status can do so. This status, RESIGNED, is for those who: (1) no longer wish to satisfy the continuing education requirements; (2) no longer wish to pay the NATABOC annual certification fee or pay the annual certified membership dues for the NATA; or (3) wish to permanently leave the profession of athletic training.

2. A certified athletic trainer who voluntarily resigns his or her certification and is therefore classified as RESIGNED, agrees not to do the following:

a) serve as a supervisor of students who are satisfying their requirements for certification eligibility;

b) serve as a model or examiner for the NATABOC certification examination; or

c) represent him or herself to the public as a practicing certified athletic trainer or use the initials "ATC" or "C.A.T" after his or her name.

3. A certified athletic trainer who voluntarily resigns his or her certified status (NATABOC status RESIGNED) will be referred to as RETIRED* with NATA and other public information purposes.

*Addendum: A certified athletic trainer that has resigned his/her certification may request retired membership status with the NATA membership department. In order to be a retired status candidate a member must have 20 years or more of membership. The request to be changed to retired status must be in writing to the membership department of NATA.

4. An individual classified as RESIGNED who fails to adhere to the above stated conditions will be subject to the NATABOC Standards of Professional Practice and Disciplinary Process.

E. Suspension Policy

The continuing Education audit is a policy of NATABOC. Its purpose is to verify compliance with the NATABOC continuing education requirements. Falsification of the continuing education report, or failure to comply with the documentation requirements may result in revocation of certification.

A random audit will occur. Certificates have 45 days to comply with the audit. Once audited, a certificant is removed from further audits for the same term.

All certificants are instructed to maintain their records for one year following the completion of a continuing education term.

Failure to Comply Within Timeframe

1. Certificants would be in violation of Standard 7 of the Standards of Professional Practice and Disciplinary Process.

[7]. Not adhering to the eligibility requirement for certification candidacy or recertification requirements and Standards of Professional Practice of the profession.

2. Letter of non-compliance with the NATABOC would be sent via procedures outlined in the Professional Practice & Disciplinary Process.

3. Professional Practice and Discipline Committee will follow the processes outlined and act on each case individually.

APPENDIX 20

State Licensure Boards

For an up-to-date list please see the NATA website at
http://www.nata.org/downloads/documents/documents.htm

ALABAMA
Alabama Board of Athletic Trainers
PO Box 11477
1274 Gregory Ave.
Montgomery, AL 36111
(334) 284-1929
Fax (334) 284-2663
Louise Porter

ARIZONA
Arizona Board of Athletic Training
5060 N 19th Ave, Ste 209
Phoenix, AZ 85015
(602) 589-6337
Fax (602) 589-8354
Mindi Brown

ARKANSAS
Arkansas Board of Athletic Training
9 Shackleford Plaza, Suite 1
Little Rock, AR 72211
(501) 228-7100
Fax (501) 228-5535
Jennifer Coleman
Jcole101456@aol.com

COLORADO
Colorado Board of Medical Examiners
1560 Broadway, Suite 1300
Denver, CO 80202
(303) 894-7690
Fax (303) 894-7692
Susan Miller

CONNECTICUT
Department of Public Health
PO Box 340308
M.S. #12 MQA
Hartford, CT 06134
(860) 509-7603
Fax (860) 509-7607
Debra Tomassone
debra.tomassone@po.state.ct.us

DELAWARE
Examining Board of Physical Therapy
Division of Professional Regulation
Cannon Bldg, Suite 203
861 Silver Lake Blvd.
Dover, DE 19904
(302) 739-4522 x206
Fax (302)739-2711
Susan Miccio
smiccio@state.de.us

FLORIDA
Florida State Health Department
Board of Athletic Trainers
4052 Bald Cypress Way, BIN C08
Tallahassee, FL 30127
(850) 245-4444 ext 3463 or (850) 245-4474
Theresa Skelton
www.doh.state.fl.us/mga/athtrain/athome.htm
Theresa_Skelton@DOH.state.fl.us

GEORGIA
Georgia Board of Athletic Trainers
237 Coliseum Drive
Macon, Georgia 31217-3858
(912) 207-1670
Fax (912) 207-1676
LaSharn Hughes, Executive Director

HAWAII
Ruth Gushiken, Executive Secretary
State of Hawaii Department of Commerce and
Consumer Affairs
Vocational Licensing Division
State Board of Physical Therapy
1010 Richards St.
Honolulu, HI 96813
(808) 586-2698

IDAHO
Idaho State Board of Medicine
1755 Westgate Dr.
PO Box 83720
Boise, ID 83720-0058
(208) 327-7000
Fax (208) 327-7005
Nancy Kerr

ILLINOIS
Dept. of Professional Regulation
Technical Assistance
096 Athletic Training
Illinois Board of Athletic Training
320 W. Washington, 3rd Floor
Springfield, IL 62786
(217) 782-8556
Fax (217) 782-7645
Cheryl Fox

INDIANA
Indiana Athletic Trainers Board
Health Professions Bureau
402 West Washington Street
Room 041
Indianapolis, IN 46204
(317) 232-2960
Fax (317) 233-4236
Barbara Buck
Bbuck@hpb.state.in.us

IOWA
Iowa Board of Athletic Training
Lucas State Office Bldg, 5th Floor
321 East 12th Street
Des Moines, IA 50319-0075
(515) 281-4401
(515) 281-3121
Roxanne Sparks

KANSAS
Kansas State Board of the Healing Arts
235 S. Topeka Blvd.
Topeka, KS 66603
(785) 296-7413
(785) 296-0852
Charlene Abbott
Cabbott@ink.org

KENTUCKY
Kentucky Board of Medical Licensure
310 Whittington Parkway, Ste. 1B
Louisville, KY 40222
(502) 429-8046
Fax (502) 429-9923
Martha Smith
Martha.smith@mail.state.ky.us

LOUISIANA
State Board of Medical Examiners
630 Camp Street
New Orleans, LA 70130
Mailing Address:
P. O. Box 30250
New Orleans, LA 70190-0250
(504) 524-6763
Fax (504) 599-0503
Carol Duchmann

MAINE
Maine Department of Professional and
Financial Regulation
Office of Licensing & Registration
Board of Athletic Trainers
35 State House Station
Augusta, ME 04333-0035
(207) 624-8624
Fax (207) 624-8637
Marlene McFadden

MASSACHUSETTS
Board of Allied Health Professions
239 Causeway St., Ste 400
Boston, MA 02214-2130
(617) 727-3071
Fax (617) 727-2669
Kimberly Hamel
kimberly.a.hamel@state.ma.us

MINNESOTA
Athletic Trainers' Advisory Council
State Board of Medical Practice
University Park Plaza
2829 University Ave. Ste 400
Minneapolis, MN 55414-3246

(612) 617-2145
Fax (612) 617-2166
Erika Oberfrank
erikao@bmp.state.mn.us

MISSISSIPPI
Mississippi State Department of Health
Office of Professional Licensure
PO Box 1700
Jackson, MS 39215-1700
(601) 987-4153
Fax (601) 987-3784
David Kweller

MISSOURI
Missouri St Board for the Healing Arts
PO Box 4
Jefferson City, MO 65102
(573) 751-0098
Fax (573) 751-3166
Karla Laughlin

NEBRASKA
Department of HHS Regulation & Licensure
PO Box 94986
Lincoln, NE 68509
(402) 471-0547
Fax (402) 471-3577
Diane Hansmeyer
Doh6151@vmhost.cdp.state.ne.us

NEW HAMPSHIRE
Office of Allied Health Professionals
2 Industrial Park Drive
Concord, NH 03301
(603) 271-8389
Fax (603) 271-6702

Veronique Soucy
Aboldus@nhsa.state.nh.us

NEW JERSEY
The Board of Medical Examiners
Athletic Training Advisory Committee
140 East Front Street, 2nd Floor
PO Box 183
Trenton, NJ 08625-0183
(609) 826-7100
Fax (609) 826-7117
Mary Lou Mattola

NEW MEXICO
Regulation & Licensing Department
Athletic Training Practice Board
PO Box 25101
Santa Fe, NM 87504
(505) 476-7100
Fax (505) 476-7094
Becky Armijo-Lakey
AthleticTrainerBoard@state.nm.us

NEW YORK
Division of Professional Licensing Serv
State Committee for Athletic Trainers
89 Washington Ave
Albany, NY 12234-1000
(518) 474-3817
Fax (518) 486-4846
Karen Anderson
Athlbd@mail.nysed.gov

NORTH CAROLINA
Board of Athletic Training Examiners
PO Box 10769
Raleigh, NC 27605

(919) 821-4980
Fax (919) 833-5743
Jim Scarborough
Scarboro@interpath.com

NORTH DAKOTA
Board of Athletic Trainers
118 Independence Ave
Bismark, ND 58503-0463
(701)255-7500
Tim McCrory, ATC

OHIO
Executive Secretary
OT, PT, AT Board
77 S. High Street, 16th Floor
Columbus, OH 43266-0317
(800) 871-1921
(614) 466-3774
Fax (614) 644-8112
Carl Gabriel Williams or Stephanie Youst
SRS_OPT_RB@ohio.gov

OKLAHOMA
Board of Medical Licensure & Supervision
Athletic Trainers Advisory Committee
PO Box 18256
Oklahoma City, OK 73154
(405) 848-6841
Fax (405) 848-8240
Kathy Plant
Osbmls@osbmls.state.ok.us
www.osbmls.state.ok.us

OREGON
Health Division Licensing Programs
Board of Athletic Trainers

700 Summer Street NE, Suite 230
Salem, OR 97310-1287
(503) 378-8667
Fax (503) 585-9114
E-mail: hdlp.mail@state.or.us
www.hdlp.hr.state.or.us
Tricia Allbritton
patricia.c.allbritton@state.or.us

PENNSYLVANIA
Bureau of Professional & Occupational Affairs
PO Box 2649
Harrisburg, PA 17105-2649
(717) 783-7134
Fax (717) 787-7769
Robert Kline
Physical@pados.dos.state.pa.us

RHODE ISLAND
Rhode Island Department of Health
Division ofProfessional Regulations
3 Capital Hill, Room 105
Providence, RI 02908
(401)222-2827 x104
(401) 222-5888
Fax (401) 222-3352
Paula Morrissey
www.health.state.ri.us/hsr/at_train.htm

SOUTH CAROLINA
SC DHEC
Division of EMS
2600 Bull St.
Columbia, SC 29201
(803) 737-7204
Fax (803) 737-7212
Jim Catoe
CatoeJC@Columb54.DHEC.state.us

SOUTH DAKOTA
South Dakota Board of Medical & Osteopathic
Examiners
1323 S. Minnesota Ave.
Sioux Falls, SD 57105
(605) 334-8343
Fax (605) 336-0270
Mitzi Turley

TENNESSEE
Board of Medical Examiners
State Department of Health
Council on Athletic Training
1st Floor, Cordell Hull Building
425 Fifth Ave. North
Nashville, TN 37247-1010
(888) 310-4650 or (615) 741-3824
Fax (615) 532-5369
Vickie Pentecost

TEXAS
Advisory Board of Athletic Trainers
1100 West 49th Street
Austin, TX 78756-3183
(512) 834-6615
Fax (512) 834-6677
Steven Mills
Stephen.mills@tah.state.tx.us
www.tdh.state.tx.us/hcqs/plc/at.htm

VERMONT
Secretary of State's Office
Office of Professional Regulation
26 Terrace St., Drawer 09
Montpelier, VT 05609-1106

(802) 828-2390
Diane Lafaille
dlafaill@sec.state.vt.us

VIRGINIA
Department of Health Professions
6606 W Broad St., 4th Floor
Richmond, VA 23230-1717
(804) 662-9900
Fax (804) 662-9114
Robert Nebiker or William Hart, MD

WEST VIRGINIA
West Virginia Department of Education
Building 6, Room 309
1900 Kanawha Boulevard East
Charleston, WV 25305-0330
(304) 558-8830
Fax (304) 558-0048
John Ray, Coordinator

WISCONSIN
Dept of Regulation & Licensing
Athletic Trainers Affiliated Credentialing Board
PO Box 8935
Madison, WI 53708-8935
(608) 266-0483
(608) 261-7083
Patrick Braatz

APPENDIX 21

Prescription Drugs by Disease/Disorder*

Reprinted with permission from Jacobs K. *Quick Reference Dictionary for Occupational Therapy.* 2nd ed. Thorofare, NJ: SLACK Incorporated; 1999.

Alcohol Withdrawal
Librium
ReVia
Valium

Alzheimer's Disease
Aricept
Cognex

Angina
Adalat
Inderal
Isoptin
Procardia

Anxiety Disorders
Benzodiazepine
Ativan
Klonopin
Valium
Xanax

Beta-Blockers
Inderal
Miscellaneous
BuSpar

Arthritis
Actron
Advil
Anaprox
Ansaid
Daypro
Feldene
Indocin
Lodine
Motrin
Naprosyn
Pediapred
Relafen
Rufen
Toradol

Asthma
Accolate
AeroBid
Alupent
Azmacort
Brethine
Intal
Lufyllin
Medrol
Nasacort

Note: The following is a list of brand name and generic drugs. Please consult each drug's literature for further information. Mention of specific products is not intended as an endorsement by the author or publisher.

Proventil
Theo-Dur
Ventolin

*Attention Deficit
Hyperactivity Disorder*
Adderall
Cylert
Dexedrine
Ritalin

Cancer
Arimidex
Cisplatin
Cytoxan
Deltasone
Efudex
Estrace
Estraderm
Medrol
Methotrexate
Orasone
Pediapred
Premarin
Tamoxifen
Taxol

Depression
Tricyclic Antidepressants
Aventyl
Elavil
Norpramin
Pamelor
Sinequan
Tofranil

*Serotonin Uptake
Inhibitors*
Paxil
Prozac
Zoloft

*Monoamine Oxidase
MAO) Inhibitors*
Lithium
Nardil
Parnate

Miscellaneous
Desyrel
Effexor
Lithium
Serzone
Vivactil
Wellbutrin

Fluid Retention
Bumex
Diamox
Diuril
Dyazide
Esidrix
Lasix
Lozol
Maxzide
Thalitone

Headache, Cluster
Calan
Depakote
Lithium
Sansert

Headache, Migraine
Amerge
Cafergot
Imitrex
Inderal
Maxalt
Midrin
Nadolol
Wygesic
Zomig

Headache, Tension
Anolor
Esgic
Fioricet
Fiorinal
Fiorinal with Codeine

Heart Attack
Atenolol
Captopril
Inderal
Lopressor
Prinivil
Tenormin
Zestril

High Blood Pressure
Accupril
Adalat
Aldomet
Altace
Calan
Catapres
Lasix
Lopressor

Lotrel
Moduretic
Norvasc
Procardia

Infection, HIV
Crixivan
Epivir
Hivid
Invirase
Norvir
Retrovir
Videx
Viramune
Zerit

Infections, Lower Respiratory Tract
Amoxil
Augmentin
Biaxin
Ceclor
Ceftin
E-Mycin
Flagyl
Ilotycin
Keflex
Pen-Vee K
Tetracycline
Zithromax

Infections, Upper Respiratory Tract
Amoxicillin with
    Clavulanate
Augmentin

Bactrin
Ceclor
Ceftin
E-Mycin
Flagyl
Keflex
Tetracycline

Inflammatory Diseases
Anaprox
Decadron Tablets
Deltasone
Medrol
Orasone
Pediapred

Insomnia
Ambien
Dalmane
Desyrel
Doral
Halcion
ProSom
Restoril

Muscle Relaxants
Flexeril
Norflex
Norgesic
Robaxin
Skelaxin
Soma
Valium

Obsessive-Compulsive Disorder
Anafranil
Luvox

Paxil
Prozac

Osteoporosis
Calcimar
Estrace
Estraderm
Fosamax
Miacalcin
Ogen
Premarin

Paget's Disease
Alendronate Sodium
Calcimar
Fosamax
Miacalcin

Pain
Acetaminophen
Anaprox
Ansaid
Cataflam
Clinoril
Darvocet-N
Darvon
Demerol
Ecotrin
Empirin with Codeine
Lorcet
Motrin
Naprosyn
Panadol
Talwin
Toradol
Voltaren

Parkinson's Disease
Artane
Benadryl
Cogentin
Eldepryl
Mirapex
Parlodel
Permax
Requip
Sinemet CR
Symmetrel
TaSmar

Sexually Transmitted Diseases
Acyclovir
Amoxil
Ceftin
Doryx
E-Mycin
Flagyl
Floxin
Minocin
Omnipen
Zonirax

Schizophrenia
Antipsychotics
Haldol
Mellaril
Risperdal
Stelazine
Thorazine

Seizure Disorders
Cerebyx
Depakote
Dilantin
Lamictal
Neurotonin
Phenobarbital
Tegretol

Ulcers, Peptic
Axid
Biaxin
Carafate
Prilosec
Tagamet
Zantac
Resources

RESOURCES

PDR Family Guide to Prescription Drugs. 6th ed. New York, NY: Three Rivers Press; 1998.

Physicians' Desk Reference. 52nd ed. Montvale, NJ: Medical Economics; 1999.

Weight and Measure Conversions

Reprinted with permission from Bottomley J. *Quick Reference Dictionary for Physical Therapy*. Thorofare, NJ: SLACK Incorporated; 2000.

English System

Linear Measure
12 inches = 1 foot
3 feet = 1 yard (0.9144 meter)
5.5 yards = 1 rod
40 rods = 1 furlong/220 yards
8 furlongs = 1 statute mile/1760 yards
5280 feet = 1 statute or land mile
3 miles = 1 league
6,076.11549 feet = 1 international nautical mile (1852 meters)

Dry Measure
2 pints = 1 quart
8 quarts = 1 peck
4 pecks = 1 bushel/2150.42 cubic inches

Angular and Circular Measure
60 seconds = 1 minute
60 minutes = 1 degree
90 degrees = 1 right angle
180 degrees = 1 straight angle
360 degrees = 1 circle

Square Measure
144 square inches = 1 square foot
9 square feet = 1 square yard

30.25 square yards = 1 square rod
160 square rods = 1 acre
640 acres = 1 square mile

Troy Weight
24 grains = 1 pennyweight
20 pennyweights = 1 ounce
12 ounces = 1 pound, Troy

Cubic Measure
1728 cubic inches = 1 cubic foot
27 cubic feet = 1 cubic yard

Liquid Measure
4 gills = 1 pint
2 pints = 1 quart
4 quarts = 1 gallon/231 cubic inches

Avoirdupois Weight
27.34375 grains = 1 dram
16 drams = 1 ounce
16 ounces = 1 pound/0.45359237 kilogram
100 pounds = 1 short hundredweight
20 short hundredweights = 1 short ton

The Metric System

Linear Measure
10 millimeters = 1 centimeter
10 centimeters = 1 decimeter
10 decimeters = 1 meter
10 meters = 1 dekameter
10 dekameters = 1 hectometer
10 hectometers = 1 kilometer

Liquid Measure
10 milliliters = 1 centiliter
10 centiliters = 1 deciliter

10 deciliters = 1 liter
10 liters = 1 dekaliter
10 dekaliters = 1 hectoliter
10 hectoliters = 1 kiloliter

Square Measure
100 square millimeters = 1 square centimeter
100 square centimeters = 1 square decimeter
100 square decimeters = 1 square meter
100 square meters = 1 square dekameter
100 square dekameters = 1 square hectometer
100 square hectometers = 1 square kilometer

Weights
10 milligrams = 1 centigram
10 centigrams = 1 decigram
10 decigrams = 1 gram
10 grams = 1 dekagram
10 dekagrams = 1 hectogram
10 hectograms = 1 kilogram
100 kilograms = 1 quintal
10 quintals = 1 ton

Cubic Measure
1000 cubic millimeters = 1 cubic centimeter
1000 cubic centimeters = 1 cubic decimeter
1000 cubic decimeters = 1 cubic meter

English and Metric Conversion

Linear Measure
1 centimeter = 0.3937 inch
1 inch = 2.54 centimeters
1 foot = 0.3048 meter
1 meter = 39.37 inches / 1.0936 yards
1 yard = 0.9144 meter
1 kilometer = 0.621 mile
1 mile = 1.609 kilometers

Square Measure
1 square centimeter = 0.1550 square inch
1 square inch = 6.452 square centimeters
1 square foot = 0.0929 square meter
1 square meter = 1.196 square yards
1 square yard = 0.8361 square meter
1 hectare = 2.47 acres
1 acre = 0.4047 hectare
1 square kilometer = 0.386 square mile
1 square mile = 2.59 square kilometers

Weight Measure
1 gram = 0.03527 ounce
1 ounce = 28.35 grams
1 kilogram = 2.2046 pounds
1 pound = 0.4536 kilogram
1 metric ton = 0.98421 English ton
1 English ton = 1.016 metric tons

Volume Measure
1 cubic centimeter = 0.061 cubic inch
1 cubic inch = 16.39 cubic centimeters
1 cubic foot = 0.0283 cubic meter
1 cubic meter = 1.308 cubic yards
1 cubic yard = 0.7646 cubic meter
1 liter = 1.0567 quarts
1 quart dry = 1.101 liters
1 quart liquid = 0.9463 liter
1 gallon = 3.78541 liters
1 peck = 8.810 liters
1 hecroliter = 2.8375 bushels